Color Your Life . . .
With Haircolor

Color Your Life . . . With Haircolor

LOUIS LICARI
with Sharon Esche

Photographs by Serge Barbeau
Illustrations by Valerie Dray and Antonio Lopez
Hair designed by Gad Cohen
Makeup by Craig Gadson

G. P. Putnam's Sons / New York

G. P. Putnam's Sons
Publishers Since 1838
200 Madison Avenue
New York, NY 10016

Copyright © 1985 by Louis Licari
All rights reserved. This book, or parts thereof,
may not be reproduced in any form without permission.
Published simultaneously in Canada by
General Publishing Co. Limited, Toronto

Library of Congress Cataloging in Publication Data

Licari, Louis, date.
   Color your life . . . with haircolor.

   1. Hair—Dyeing and bleaching.   I. Esche,
Sharon, date. II. Title.
TT973.L53   1985   646.7 '242   84-24854
ISBN 0-399-13021-7

Printed in the United States of America

   2   3   4   5   6   7   8   9   10

Design by Lynn Braswell

ACKNOWLEDGMENTS

Special thanks to our assistants Kathy Galotti, Joel Warren, Patricia Browne, and especially Steve Sanna, who was a driving force in the completion of this book.

Special credits go to the following:

The Ford Model Agency and Ford models Betsy Cameren, Toni DeMarco, Ty Hendrick, Lynn Pedola, Donna Sexton, and Roseanne Vela.

Elite Model Agency and Elite models Janelle Brady, Alisha Das, Gabrielle, Jill Goodacre, Heidi Kay, Cara Leigh, Sharon Middendorf, Hunter Reno, Kathy Schaer, Tara Shannon, and Jen Yarrow.

Beth Ann Model Agency and Beth Ann model Danny.

Zoli Model Agency and Zoli models Margaret Donohoe and Susi Guilder.

Click Model Agency and Click model Lauren Helm.

Nina Blanchard Model Agency and Nina Blanchard model Gina Oliveri.

Also our thanks to the models Frank Ganley and Suzanne Jeffers.

Special thanks to Phyllis Klein, Director of Public Relations at Clairol; Amy Tannenbaum for jewelry styling; Jewelry by Galleria Cano, Trump Tower; and Lori Goldstein for fashion styling.

Fashion credits given to: Berek; Blythe & Blythe; Marla Buck; Dalton; Patricia Field; Fiorucci; Good As Gold; Betsey Johnson; Keiko; Anne Klein II; Kenneth J. Lane; Marcasiano; Towels by Martex; Rebecca Moses; Giorgio Sant' Angelo; Tee Shirts by Swipes for Ithaca Industries, Inc.; Tous Les Caleçons; and Patricia Underwood.

*To Charles Booth, and La Coupe, Inc.,
who believed in Louis Licari
and
Modern Haircolor from the beginning.*

Contents

Modern Haircolor:
Your Most Important Fashion Accessory   15

1   The Excitement of Today's Haircolor   23

Looking and Feeling Better
"Paying Off" Professionally
Haircolor Is Good for Your Hair
Fabulous Fashion Effects: The Choice Is Yours
The Three Cs of Beautiful Hair: Cut, Color, and Condition

2 Helping You Make the Color Decision 39

When to Think About Coloring Your Hair
Haircolor "Facelifts" to Minimize Facial Flaws
Getting Familiar With Color Talk
Turning Terms into Techniques
Choosing the Right Color
Salon vs. At-Home Haircoloring
Take an Objective Look: Final Considerations

3 Salon Haircoloring 59

When You Need a Professional Haircolorist
How to Find the Right Colorist
The Cross-Over Clientele Generation

4   The Wonderful World of At-Home Haircoloring: *69*
　　　　The Basics

Determining the Right Type of Product
Reading the Box
The Patch Test
The Strand Test
Setting Up for Haircolor
Before You Begin . . . Some Final Thoughts

5   "How-to" At-Home Techniques   *85*

Applying All Haircolor . . . Where to Begin and End
Temporary Color Application
Semipermanent Color Application
Permanent Color Application
Fine Basic Highlighting Using a Cap
Hair Painting
Tie-Dyeing
Color Blocking
How to Lighten Eyebrows

6	Caring for Color-Treated Hair	119

Valuable Hair Care Tips
Conditioning
Special At-Home Recipes
The New Freedom of Modern Haircolor

7	"Dull-to-Dazzling" Haircolor Makeovers	129

Gabrielle: Dull-to-Shining Blond
Toni: Turning a Great Cut into a Great Look With Highlights
Lynn: "Blah" Brown to Warm Blond
Heidi: Ordinary-to-Golden Highlighted Brown
Alisha: No-Life Brown to Bouncy Brunette
Kathy: "No-Color" Hair to Rich, Coppery Auburn
Susan: Turning Gray Strands into Fabulous Highlights
Janelle: Dull Blond to the Look of a Summer of Sun

8   Haircolor for Men   *139*

The Modern Haircolor Revolution
When to Think About Haircolor
Popular Haircolor Options
Haircolor Q & A
How-to Haircolor Techniques
Beards, Mustaches, and Sideburns

Be the Best You Can Be . . .
With Haircolor   *153*

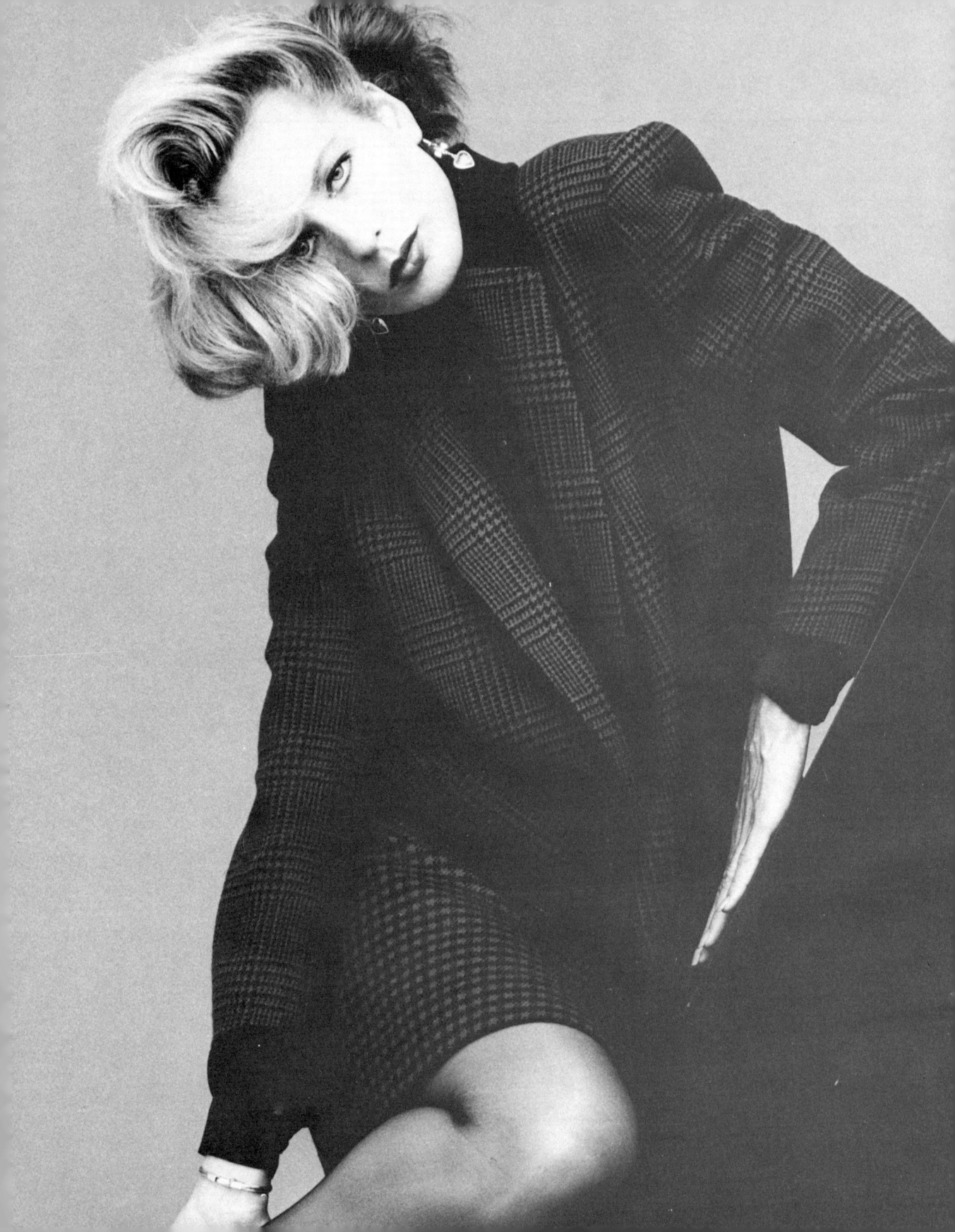

Modern Haircolor: Your Most Important Fashion Accessory

There has never been so much fashion excitement around haircolor as there is today. Haircolor is described as the newest cosmetic because it does for the hair what makeup does for the face. It creates a beautiful, shining, translucent finish for the hair, plays up your skin tones, brings out your eye color, and brightens your entire appearance.

There's no doubt that haircolor can take you from dull to dazzling in literally minutes. When your haircolor is right, you actually need less makeup. Your own natural coloring just comes shining through.

It's true that women have been coloring their hair for years. But now, modern haircolor has sent women flocking to salons and drugstore shelves for at-home products to discover the many fashion options haircolor has in store for them.

What's all the new excitement around haircolor? Unlike haircoloring in years past, modern haircolor is fun and fashionable, as well as easy to do and to maintain. Accenting your hair is as simple as buying a new blusher or lipstick. It also will make a wonderful difference in your life. Ask any one of the thirty-five million women who already color their hair . . . and color their lives.

When it comes right down to it, *you* are the "modern" in modern haircolor. Until now, you may have colored your hair to cover up "defects" such as gray. Now you can use haircolor to play up your assets, like using eye shadow or lipstick for color accent.

Haircolor has actually become your most important fashion accessory because we clearly can see the overall difference it makes in our total image or "personality." When our haircolor looks beautiful, we come alive from head to toe. When it appears rather dull and uninspiring, we downplay ourselves unnecessarily.

Unfortunately, when it comes to fashion, many women think from the neck down. They spend so much money on fabulous clothes, shoes, handbags, and jewelry that they fail to pay any attention to what's *above* those beautiful shoulders. Remember, haircolor affects our fashion image, too; the right blend of lights and tones in the hair *wakes up* the fabrics we wear. When considering total color balance—coordinating the colors of our clothing with our hair and makeup—we can see how our darker clothes cry out for a contrast of lights in the hair. The more vivid colors, like reds, blues, and yellows, all call for some sparkle or brightness in our haircolor. Likewise, whites, beiges, creams, and other neutrals look more opulent when our haircolor is rich. Dull hair minimizes the appearance of our clothes, but dazzling hair sets them off beautifully.

As a professional haircolorist, I have learned that every woman has a haircolor fantasy or a secret haircolor personality. You, too, may discover that you've always wanted to be a blonde, a redhead, or perhaps a striking brunette. Many women have turned their fantasies into reality. Even if it's just adding a few highlights or subtly enhancing your own natural shade, modern haircolor offers you dozens of easy options to be whatever you want to be.

My theory that haircolor "colors your life" is proven with every woman who walks out of my salon. If I viewed every client as a "case study" in the impact of haircolor on our lives, I could share thousands of happy stories with you. But now that I have you thinking of your own haircolor, let me share some important thoughts I always share with my clients.

I want you to know that there are two easy avenues to more beautiful hair. One is to color your hair at home, which is so easy it's fun. There's no guesswork involved—haircolor manufacturers have done the hard thinking for us. They now offer products that are virtually foolproof. No-fuss, total-control haircoloring with predictable results—that's what modern haircolor is all about.

The other avenue to more beautiful hair is salon haircoloring. There are many special effects or more complicated techniques that your professional haircolorist does best. Modern product technology has also helped professionals; they now have the optimal ranges of fabulous, natural-looking shades to custom blend just for the individual.

If you are among those thirty-five million women (the numbers are growing all the time) already coloring their hair, perhaps you're ready for something new. No one's hair should remain the same year after year. In fact, I recommend some sort of subtle color change every season along with updating the shape of your cut. Whether you're ready for a subtle change or something more dramatic, I'll show you some new fashion options and new personal color formulas to consider.

So many people ask me if everyone should color their hair. Deep down, professionally and personally, my answer is *yes*. I really believe there is something "more" for everyone. No matter how gorgeous your haircolor, even a few highlights can make a wonderful difference.

I made up a slogan that sums up my feelings about haircolor: "How do you make a beautiful woman more beautiful . . . with haircolor, of course." I have practiced this philosophy on many of the most beautiful women in the world who have become my clients—famous cover girls, top runway fashion models, exquisite celebrities, and glamorous film personalities. Many careers have been helped greatly by achieving the right haircolor for an individual look.

Since the world is not made up only of movie stars and models, I want to state forcefully that every woman has her own incredible beauty. Haircolor helps that beauty to emerge in full bloom, and lets that great colorful personality come shining through!

Haircolor has so many benefits in store for you. *Color Your Life* will help you discover just how beneficial and fun haircolor can be. Whether you try coloring your hair at home or add haircoloring to your salon services, I really want you to get started doing something I know you're going to love. You'll wonder why you didn't try it sooner!

Get ready to be the best you can be!

Louis Licari

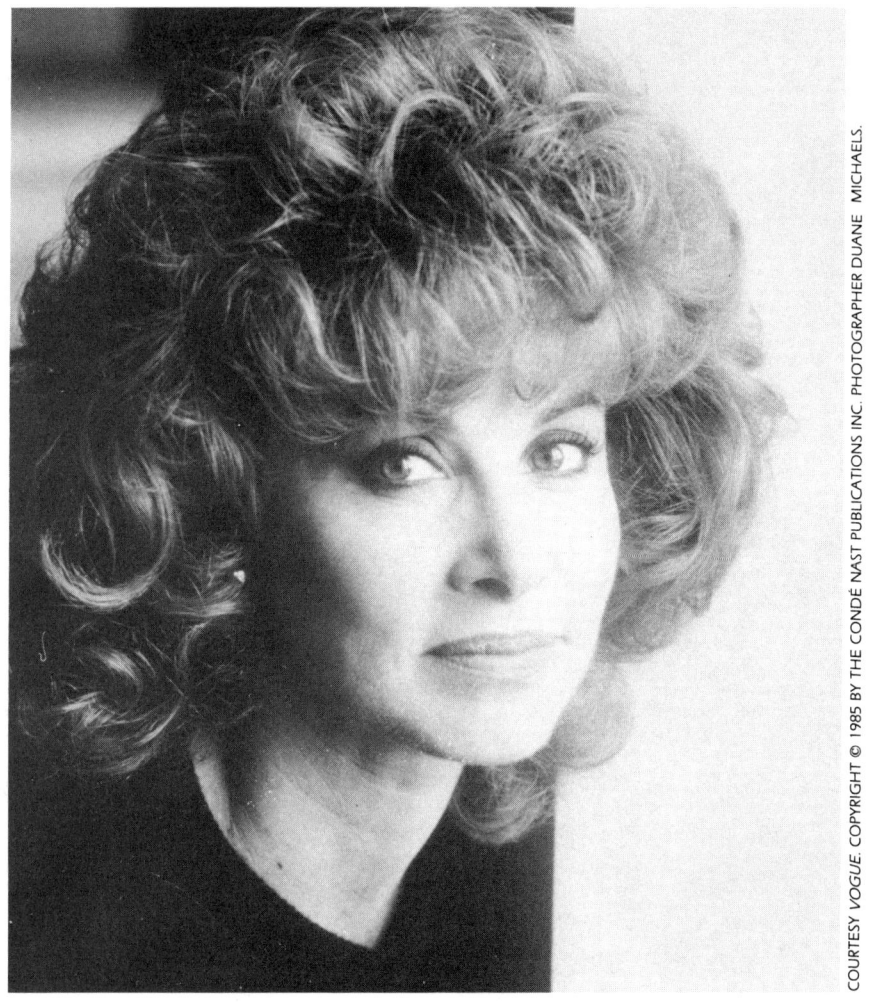

Stefanie Powers—a classic example of how a beautiful woman can be made even more beautiful . . . with just a touch of color. The famous star of "Hart to Hart" has appeared in more than twenty-seven films and a variety of successful television series. She is a woman on the go and always manages to look sleek and "pulled together" despite her incredible schedule. Her haircolor is definitely part of her stunning total image—a light, golden, warm brown. It's a beautiful combination with her fair freckled complexion and those gorgeous earth-toned clothes she loves to wear.

*Color Your Life . . .
With Haircolor*

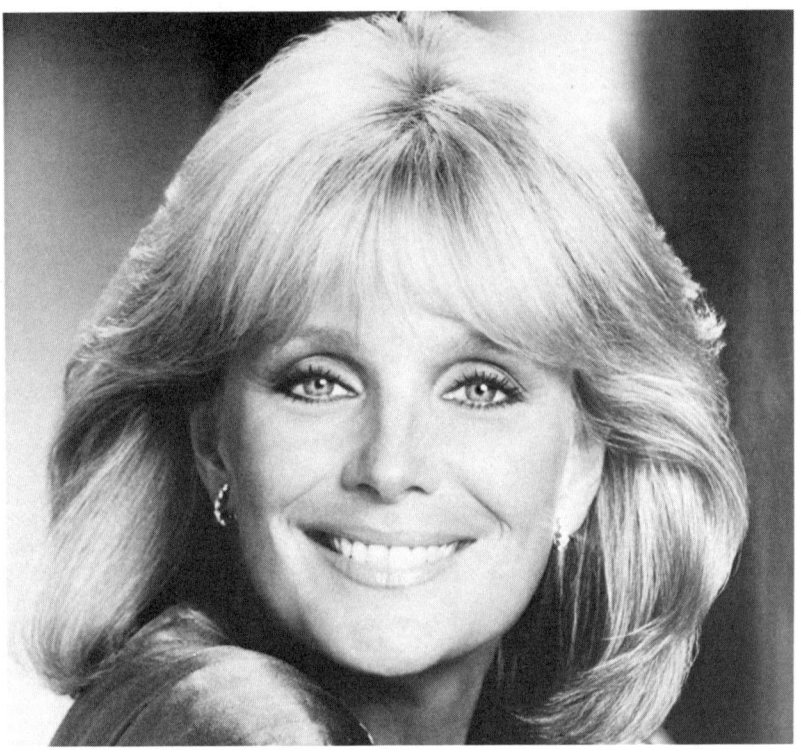

One person who exemplifies haircolor's overall positive effects is Linda Evans, the talented star of "Dynasty," the beauty in Clairol's haircolor commercials and an all-around lovely lady both personally and professionally. Haircolor certainly has colored her life and she's the first one to admit it.

"I had this horrible mousy brown hair, that dingy sort of color that always photographed a little darker. At this time, things weren't going well . . . perhaps it was the '50s; that was a very clumsy decade. I didn't think I was very pretty."

That, of course, was the Linda Evans of years past—but look at her now! She's a stunning blonde whose hair is just the right shade for her glowing personality. I would describe her as a one-process blonde with highlights especially around the face to accent the skin tones and eye color.

Linda sums it all up: "I only began to see myself as extra-attractive when I was asked to lighten my hair for a TV pilot early in my career. I was finally delighted to be acknowledged for my beauty as well as my brains."

Chapter 1

The Excitement of Today's Haircolor

Looking and Feeling Better

When we improve something about our appearance, we *automatically* feel better about ourselves. This is simply a law of nature.

The all-over positive emotional impact of improving our hair's appearance ranks high "up there" with losing weight, buying new clothes, working out to stay fit, and even getting a great new haircut. The results are all the same; you look better, feel younger, act more confident, and experience a wonderful psychological boost!

The rediscovery, of sorts, of haircoloring has a lot to do with doing good things for your self-image that are easy, fun and fast. The modern haircolor revolution has hit all age groups and both sexes full force.

Teenage girls are tie-dyeing their braids and ponytails. College guys are "suntanning" their hair with "surfer" highlights. Male executives are turning their dull, graying hair into a distinguished blend of highlights against their natural color. Women are creating new fashion effects by coloring only sections of their hair and trying out a temporary mood color for a particular night's party.

Modern haircoloring is so versatile; it can appear classic or contemporary, but always beautiful. Looking terrific with haircolor is as simple as *one, two, three!*

"Paying Off" Professionally

Looking and feeling better about ourselves is the greatest benefit haircolor has to offer. Beyond that, changing our haircolor can also make a big difference in more tangible things like the amount of money we can make on the job.

Positive first impressions on job interviews have a lot to do with haircolor. We all know that more women than ever are reentering the work force: Young mothers are seeking the additional family income, older women whose children have grown are searching for new interests, and even grandmothers are looking for ways to utilize their time. Regardless of why women work, their haircolor actually makes a difference in whether they get the job, and exactly how much salary they're offered.

Read the following headline that announces a major city study of personnel managers and employment counselors and you'll be as surprised as I was. . . .

NEW STUDY DOCUMENTS ECONOMIC ADVANTAGES OF LOOKING GOOD

Dr. Judith Waters, Professor of Psychology at Fairleigh Dickinson in New Jersey, conducted this study which was sponsored by Clairol and executed under her supervision by Market Facts, Inc., an independent research organization. It involved 120 personnel managers and employment counselors in New York, Chicago, and Los Angeles.

These individuals were shown either "before" or "after" pictures of women between the ages of twenty-five and fifty-five. The "before" photos were taken as the women actually looked. No attempt was made to make them appear unattractive. Before the "after" photos were taken, each woman had a series of subtle changes made in her haircolor, hairstyle, and makeup. They were changes any woman could easily maintain herself.

The study found that even subtle changes definitely influence employability. This is particularly true at entry-level positions where the potential employer must choose between equally qualified applicants. Furthermore, "after" photographs prompted starting salary offers of 8 to 20 percent higher due to the applicant's sharper appearance.

"While the social advantages of attractiveness have long been documented, this was the first study done on the effect in dollars and cents of looking good in the work situation.

"Since participants did not know the intended focus of the study, it is interesting how often appearance was cited in evaluating the applicant. Comments such as 'Excellent appearance—corporate image' or 'Not very neat. I wouldn't hire her

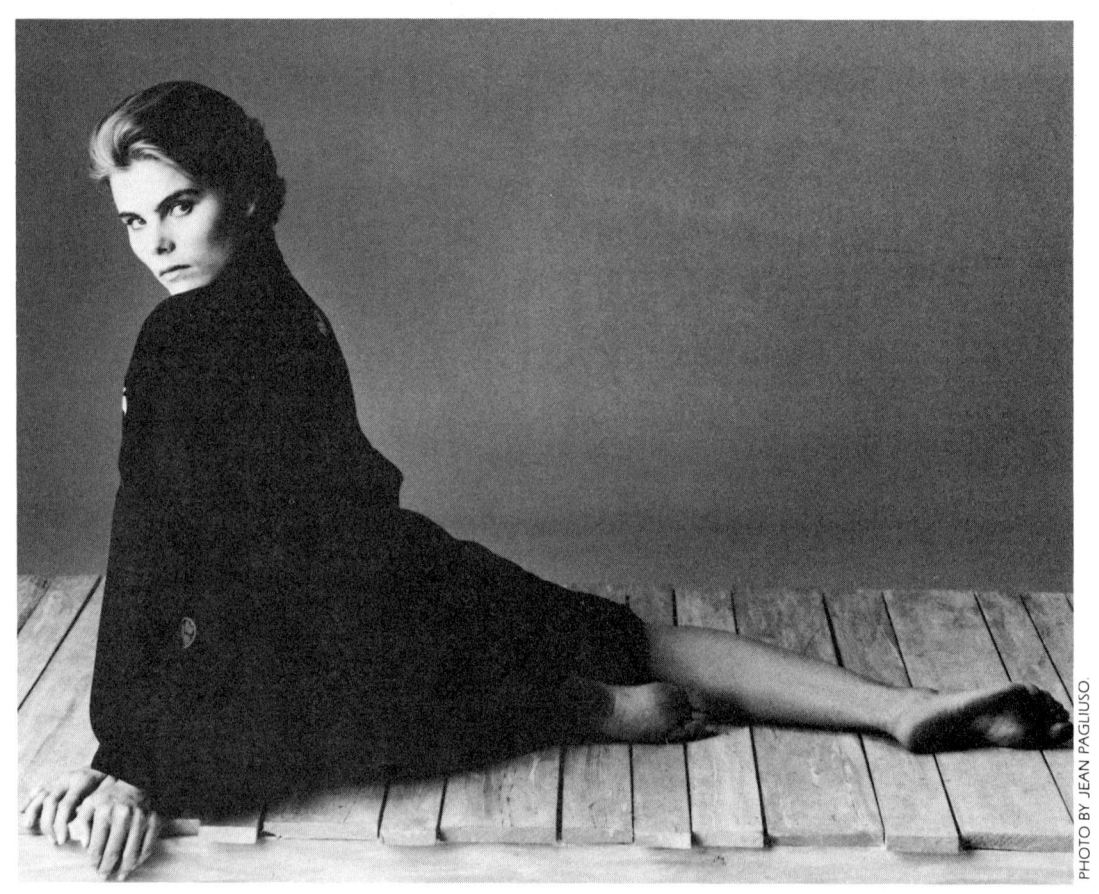

PHOTO BY JEAN PAGLIUSO

Haircolor certainly plays an important role in the professional life of Mariel Hemingway. I think of her as a natural beauty who takes on the look of the seasons—the sporty, outdoor type whose makeup, clothes, and haircolor really suit her lifestyle. But when it comes to being a film star, the right haircolor really helps her "get into" the character she's playing.

"I love the look of the California blonde—really athletic looking with natural sunny highlights in her hair. This was what I played in Personal Best—when my haircolor was adjusted to suit the role, I felt the character of this role. Haircolor definitely affects my attitude."

Mariel recalls that for a part she had in a play "I had to put on a red wig . . . it was terrific being a redhead."

even though it seems like she is qualified in what she does'" were heard frequently, Dr. Waters reports.

"It boils down to a question of self-image," says Dr. Waters. "The implication is that if she cares about herself, she probably relates better to others."

According to Dr. Waters, the findings are good news to the thousands of women seeking jobs, since appearance is the easiest attribute to improve. "It can take years to improve skills. Appearance can be improved in hours or minutes."

It literally pays to improve your appearance.

Haircolor Is Good for Your Hair

Women are usually surprised at the fact that haircolor offers other benefits to hair beyond improving its color. I'm sure you have heard the following types of questions from time to time, but I'll bet haircolor was never your answer until now.

Here's a question I am asked quite often . . . and my answer always opens a few eyes.

Q. *My hair looks dull and dry . . . how can I put the shine back into it?*

A. With haircolor, of course!

The traditional answer is to use a conditioner and moisturizers. But haircolor also improves the condition and texture of the hair; manufacturers have created gentle formulas that have conditioners built right into them. Today's color formulas help to nurture and fortify the hair as well as color it—with enriching ingredients like collagen protein, lanolin, and silk proteins. These all help to create luster and manageability plus beautiful color tones and nuances.

The following is another "eye-opener":

Q. *How can I add more body to my fine, limp hair?*

A. With haircolor, of course.

Modern haircolor products are so advanced technologically that they can actually add body and full texture to the hair. This is because they contain such ingredients as aloe vera to add smoothness to the hair shaft, panthenol (vitamin B) for fuller texture and volume, cationic silicone for incredible added volume, and vitamin E and hydraulized protein to maintain the hair's natural moisture. All these ingredients "plump" out the hair for more body.

Fabulous Fashion Effects: The Choice Is Yours

Whether you're a blonde, redhead, brunette or something in between, many fashion moods can be created with modern haircolor.

The choice is yours . . . it's like going into your favorite boutique or makeup counter and picking whatever appeals to you at the time. Special-effects haircolor is your way to "shop around" for fashion for the hair . . . and you'll love this new experience.

Later on, I'll show you how much fun it is to create these special fashion effects for any occasion, but take the time now to review your choices. These are just some of the many effects you can create at home or with the help of a professional haircolorist. Just let your imagination go . . . you'll never think of haircolor the same way again!

Color Blocking   This is an easy way to color just sections of your hair. Imagine a short or chin-length cut, and then think about how interesting it would look if you made the sides and the back a bit lighter or darker than the rest of your hair. Think of color blocking as creating beautiful shadows by *blocking out* the section you want to make darker or lighter. It's an intriguing cosmetic fashion effect for your hair.

Tie-dyeing   Remember those beautiful tie-dyed effects we loved on T-shirts, jeans, and handbags? Now our hair can show those same fun color blends in virtually any array of color we choose. I recommend this for teenagers with longer hair who are always looking for something new. Wrap up your hair as sketched on pages 112–13, spray on the color of your dreams, and then let your hair down. Voilà . . . tie-dyed hair.

Illusions   You can create just about any illusion with haircolor. With the creative use of highlighting, for instance, you can make one area the focal point—or improve upon a facial feature you've always been self-conscious about. For example, throwing more light around the face with highlights makes a small forehead appear slightly bigger. By framing your face with a color lighter than your own, you can also minimize facial wrinkles and/or make skin tones more complementary.

See chapter 2 for more information on minimizing facial flaws.

Glazing Glazing your hair achieves rich, shining, translucent color using permanent haircoloring. Glazing or glossing your hair is a simple matter of whipping up a blend of color and shampoo (called a soap cap) and applying it all over your hair. Just a few minutes later, rich tones will emerge—and your hair will have a highly polished sheen that will make any redhead, blonde, or brunette come alive.

Silhouettes Many hairstyles have beautiful shapes; they almost cry out for someone to come along and "outline" them for a great fashion accent. With a fine brush, color or light can delicately trace just the surface of the whole head, or perhaps only the soft wave patterns or the "circles" of curls, or even just the interesting edges of the bangs. Here, you're using color to literally show off shapes—the silhouette of your style.

Two-way Color Wear your hair forward and you're a rich "carmelized" brown—throw your hair back and you're a butterscotch blonde. You can have duo-color personality depending on your mood and how you wear your hair that day! Any combination of two colors can be yours. Two-way color provides color and style that can change totally with a flick of your hairbrush.

Brush-on Blushers Blushers . . . for your hair? Of course! It's all part of today's concept of haircolor as a cosmetic for your hair. Now, you can add a blush of color at the temples, to the bangs or to the top section with a makeup brush and packed powder color that looks just like a blusher kit. Depending on your haircolor and skin tone, brush on peach or amber, tawny or mauve, copper or bronze, or pick from one of many more choices.

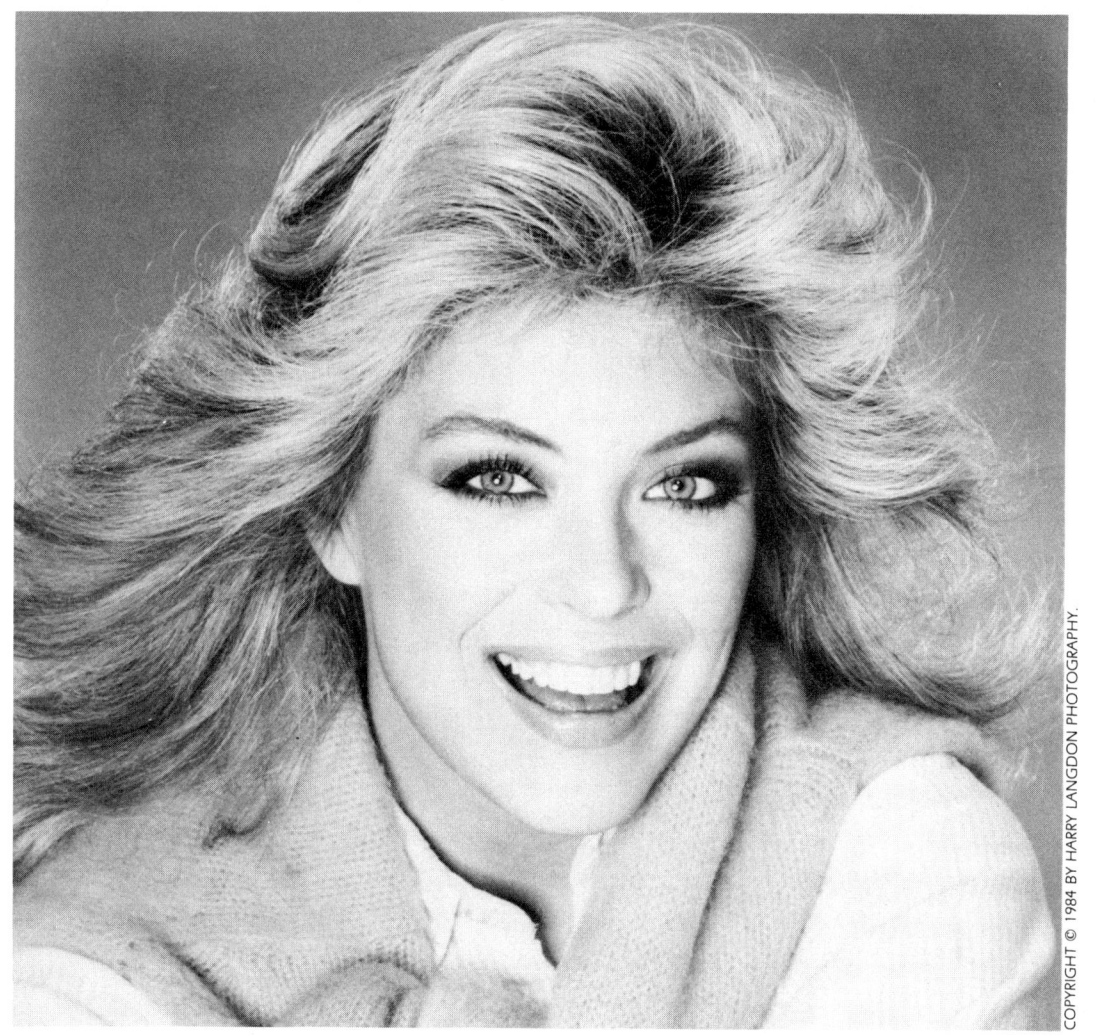

I think that Lydia Cornell is so vibrant and beautiful, she could never be "Too Close for Comfort" for me. (Sorry for the pun . . . I couldn't resist.) This bright young television star is an excellent example of silhouetting, one of today's fabulous fashion techniques. Lots of sunny highlights follow the line of her hairstyle, creating a bright allover glow. Her hair certainly looks "kissed" by the California sun.

Says Lydia: "I definitely have a blonde personality, and highlights just bring my personality out even more."

Nite-Glittering I am always fascinated when I see those fabulous glitter colors on display for the hair. You see just about any color you can think of in little "sprinkle on" pots of magical glitter—hot pinks, electric blues, passionate purples, emerald greens, plus gold, silver, and copper. Glitter colors come in spray cans and gels too—apply them to your hair in any dose that is "you." Even a few glitters will make you look incredible under the night lights.

Chameleon Colors Definitely for the woman of many moods, this special fashion effect allows your hair to reflect a variety of lights and tones. Looked at one way, your hair may reflect golden red; from another angle, it will appear more golden blond or have richer, coppery tones.

Graffiti Colors Inspired by the street artists of New York, this is definitely a trendy new look of brighter colors that has become an art form for the hair. It's achieved by using spray-on colors, applied with either a particular design in mind or any old fun way that inspires you at the time. The colors are temporary and wash out—great for a party!

Party Gels For a sleek "wet" look that temporarily enriches your haircolor, gels are to be smoothed on to the hair depending on your cut. They help to mold and hold your hair while adding desired color tones.

The Three Cs of Beautiful Hair: Cut, Color, and Condition

There's no doubt about it: When the cut, color, and condition of your hair are ideal, something wonderful happens—your

The Excitement of Today's Haircolor

hair looks gorgeous. I call this "the three Cs of beautiful hair." When all three coexist on one head, you can't help but go from dull to dazzling.

CUT

Starting with the right cut or look for you is the first vital step for beautiful hair. Your professional stylist will create the cut that really works for your individual features and type of hair. Shaping up your hair should always precede color.

Try to be very open to new styling ideas from your hairdresser. If you have worn your hair the same old way for years, go for an exciting change.

COLOR

The second vital step is achieving beautiful color. This is what actually turns your great cut into a great "look." Color should always be thought of as light and dark contrasts in the hair. By adding softer, lighter shades or deeper, warmer tones to your own natural color, you can create the interesting contrasts that make your haircut look twice as beautiful.

In fact, when your hair has lots of light and darker tones it looks very natural. This effect actually mimics the hair we had as children—all those natural lights and nuances that have dulled over the years. Study a child's hair and you'll understand what I mean.

You can also color your hair strategically in sections or areas that accent your cut. There are many simple ways to do this, whether hair is short, chin-length, or shoulder-length. I often suggest highlighting according to the direction of the cut. You

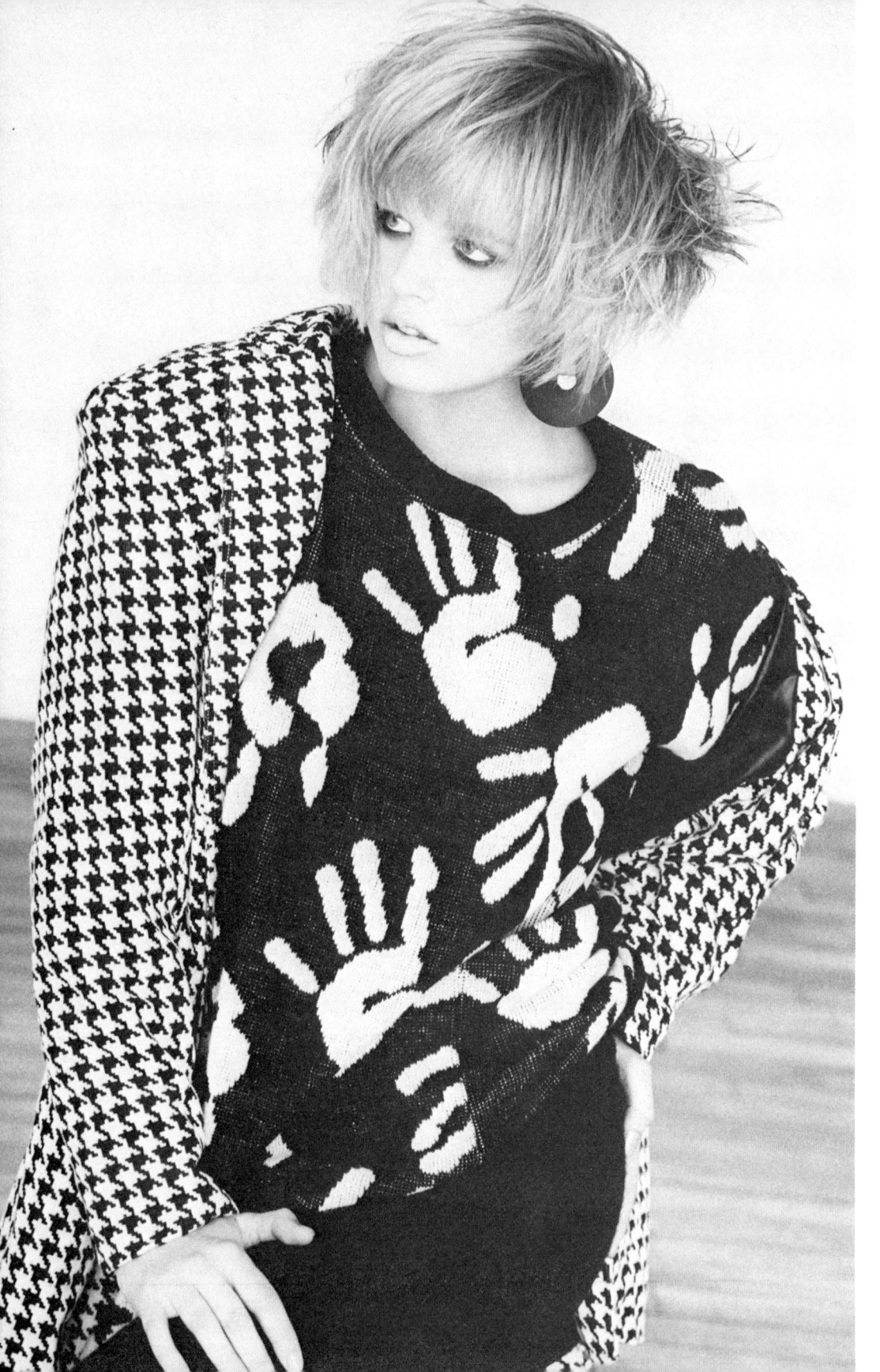

Opposite page: Lighter tones add interesting contrasts to your cut.

When highlighting follows the direction of a hairstyle, it can turn a great cut into a great look.

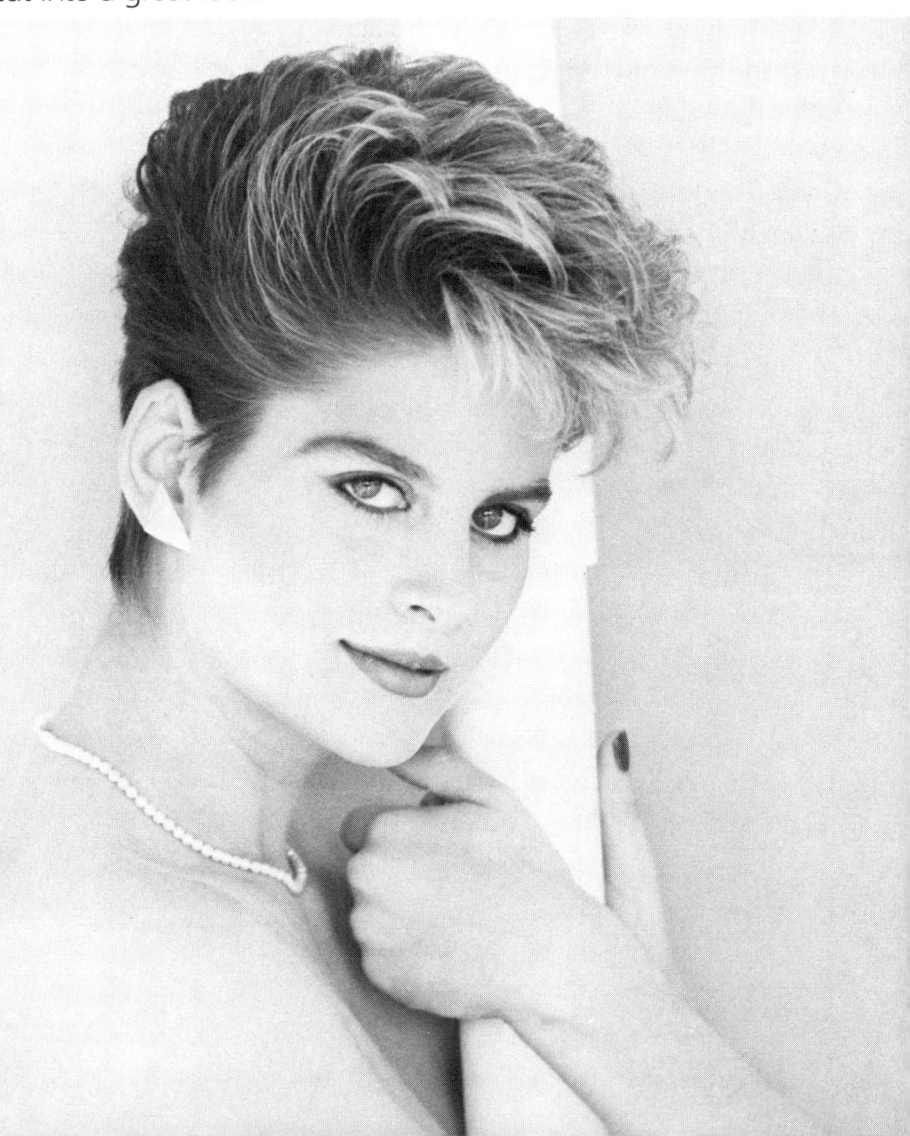

When your cut, color, and condition really work together you go from "pretty"...

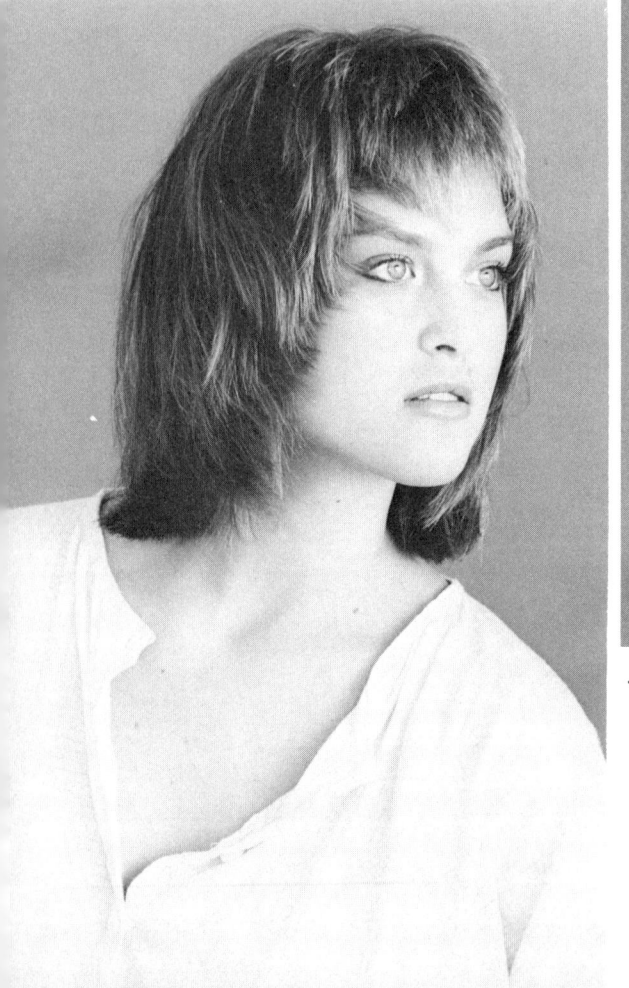

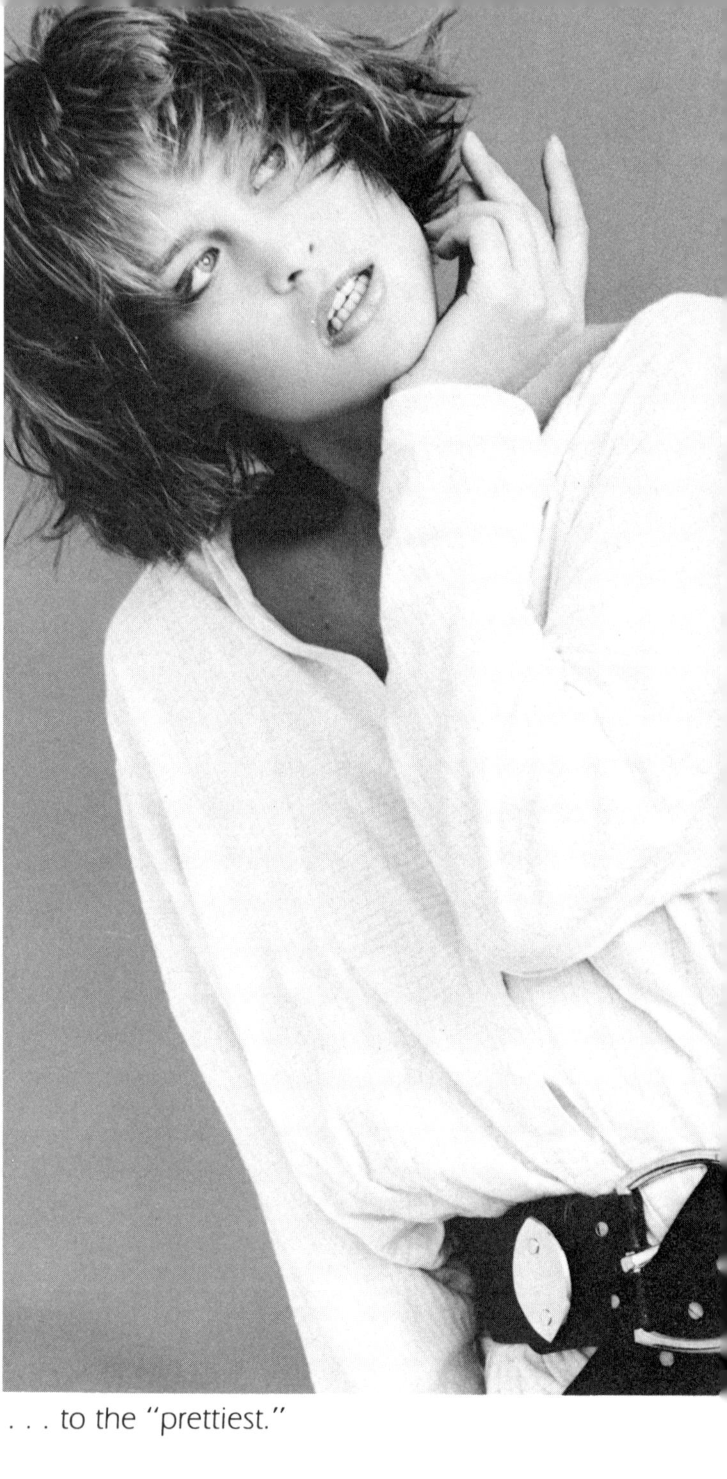

... to the "prettiest."

may want to highlight only a small section of your style for added emphasis. Or, you may want to give yourself allover color accent with haircolor either lighter or darker than your own.

One technique for accenting, called color contouring, is a way to use highlights to create motion and direction in the hair by following the natural lines of the cut.

Face-framing is another effective technique. It's a beautiful way of creating highlights only around the facial area to bring out eye color and accent skin tones.

Another technique, called tipping, is a way to outline curls and waves with either highlights or color that complements your own color. All these techniques are forms of highlighting, which is detailed further in chapter 5.

CONDITION

Now, you'll want to keep that cut and color looking in superb shape every single day. It is important to establish a regular haircare regimen. This should include an instant conditioning or remoisturizing rinse after every shampoo, plus a deep-penetrating conditioning treatment one to two times monthly depending on your hair's needs. For more conditioning information for color-treated hair, refer to chapter 6.

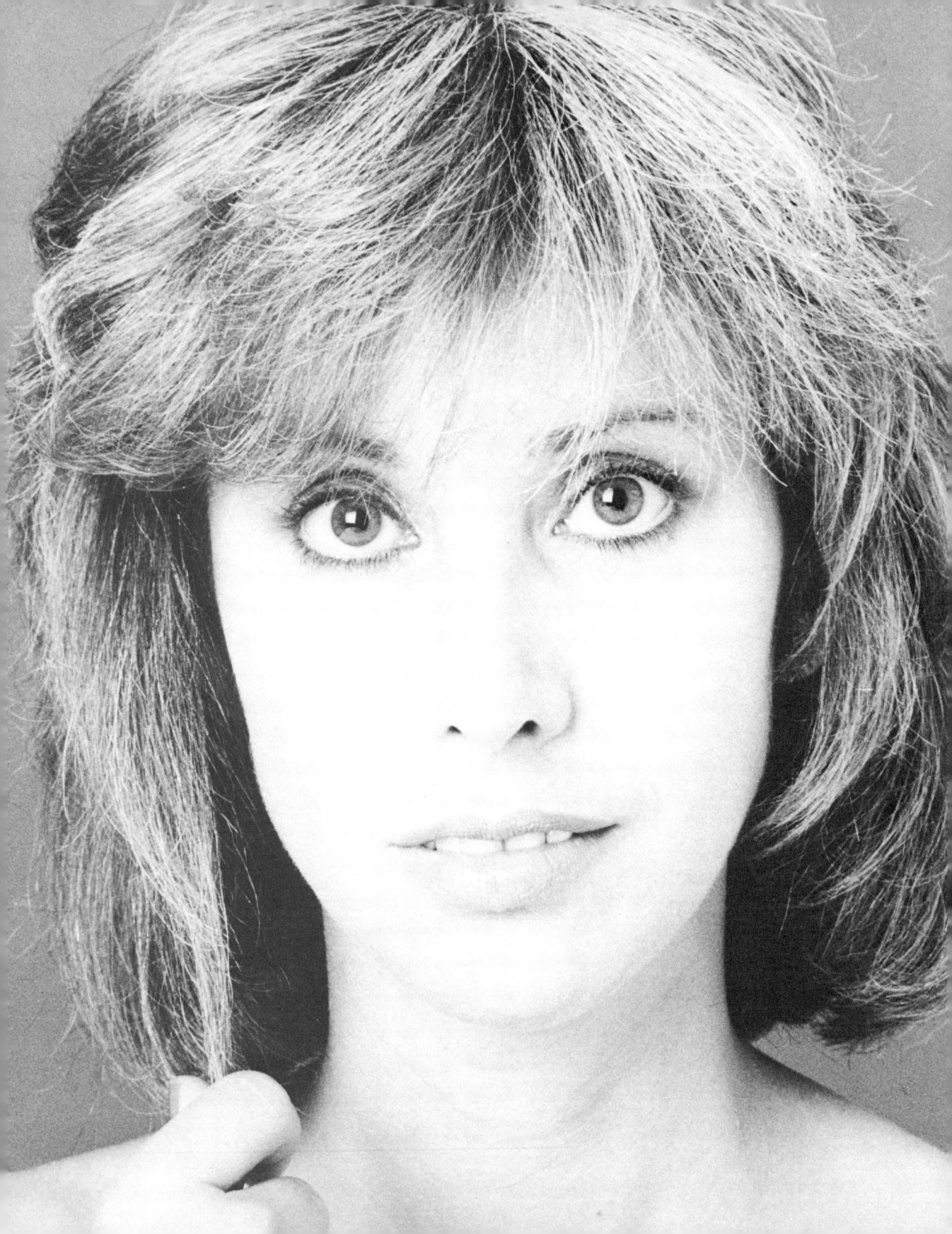

Chapter 2

Helping You Make the Color Decision

When to Think About Coloring Your Hair

I personally believe that when a woman starts to even *think* about haircoloring, she's probably ready then and there! In fact, I'll carry this one step further; there isn't a woman who *doesn't* want to color her hair in some way. It's often a secret desire that only needs to be brought out.

One dead giveaway to when a woman is ready for color is directly related to her makeup. Many women begin to wear more makeup as they get older; actually they need haircoloring to liven up dull, fading skin tones. A general rule to follow is: The more correct your haircolor, the less makeup you will need to wear as you mature. This is because haircolor gives you a generally brighter look. Natural pink skin tones can be brought out, peaches and cream complexions are made more vibrant.

Women with olive-toned complexions can look tanner or more bronze by getting a few highlights in their hair.

There are also several key points in life when thoughts about haircolor actually do surface, and it can be for the most diverse reasons. For example, most women reach a point, around the age of thirty, when their natural haircolor has dulled and a few gray strands start to show up around the hairline. At this time they may want to return to "what they once were" or try something "they have always wanted to be." Haircolor, of course, is the answer. Research shows that this is the lady who is responsible for most of the total haircolor sales today, as well as at-home products and salon haircolor services.

During emotional times, like going through a divorce, so many women come in to see me at the salon. They definitely need an emotional lift and they're smack dab in the middle of rethinking their entire lives. They're feeling insecure about their appearances, yet still are aggressive and open enough to try something new. Haircolor is the answer.

There are also those "once in a lifetime" events when women focus on their appearance and rethink their total image. These include important job changes, being the mother of the bride, and having your first baby, among other such special events. I recommend haircolor as the most perfect, fastest psychological boost. It works every time!

Thanks to modern haircolor, women who want to try something new will turn to haircolor rather than a new haircut to create some excitement. Temporary colors allow women to try a new look for a special occasion to go with a new dress and different shoes. Or, they may simply feel in need of an image update when they start to feel a bit dull.

Though no one really talks about the male influence on

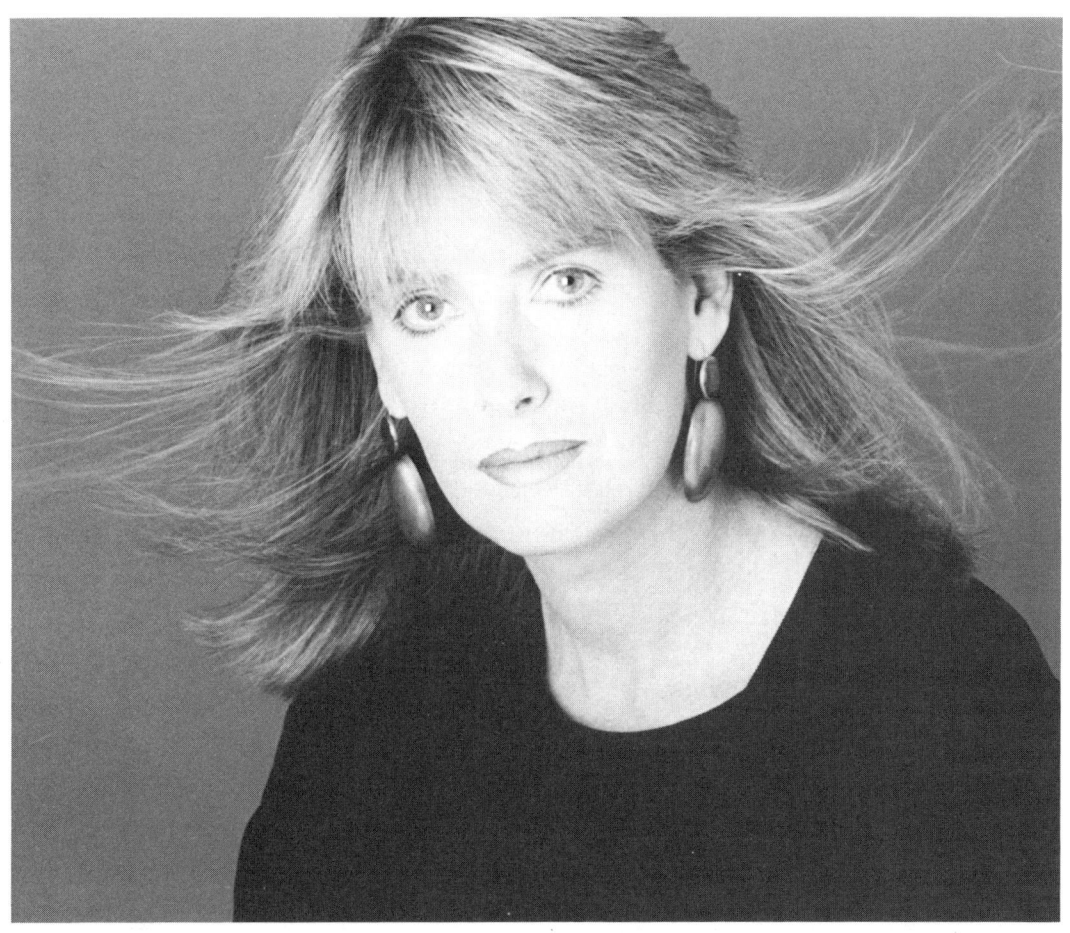

Vogue *Beauty Editor Andrea Quinn Robinson feels women of all ages use haircolor for a variety of reasons:*

"In their twenties, women use haircolor to help them look more sophisticated for their early careers. In their thirties, they look for a change and use haircolor to achieve that change. In their forties, women notice their graying hair and then decide whether to change it or go with it—haircolor can help them whatever they decide."

A beautiful sunlit blonde whose shade complements her fair, pink-toned complexion and gentle green eyes, Andrea loves the look of highlights that frame her face so naturally.

haircolor (as if it were taboo), I, nevertheless, will share a personal observation. Women used to live in dire fear of "What will my husband say?" when they "tampered" with the color of their hair. As a result, women wore their hair practically the same way from the moment they married on through the rest of their lives. Now, a woman colors her hair for her own satisfaction—to please herself and satisfy her own curiosity and very natural sense of self-exploration. If her husband or boyfriend loves it, that's great. If he doesn't, he'll love you anyway. Besides, what man could argue against playing up your natural beauty to the max? The change can be as subtle or as dramatic as you want.

In fact, haircoloring appears so natural these days, that the man in your life may just notice you're looking wonderful . . . somehow better. He may not even realize that haircolor, per se, had anything to do with it!

The last and most recognized reason for coloring your hair is to look younger. This has long been the traditional reason for women secretly using haircolor—the constant quest for shaving ten years off their looks. But this has changed with the modern woman, although looking younger remains a driving force. Women today like who they are, no matter their age. They use haircolor to enhance who and what they are—not to cover up. I call that coloring your hair for all the right reasons.

Haircolor "Facelifts" to Minimize Facial Flaws

Believe it or not, haircolor actually can be used to minimize facial flaws—another reason for coloring your hair. Like a cos-

Helping You Make the Color Decision

metic, it can play up or play down features that need some corrective camouflaging. We can use haircoloring exactly as we use our blusher and eye shadows for cosmetic contouring that really makes a difference in how we look. Haircolor can create beauty illusions in our favor.

Remembering that our haircolor goes hand in hand with our haircut, it's important to get the best style for your individual features. Then haircolor can accomplish two important things: Accent the shape of your cut and the shape of your face. Here are some expert tricks of the trade, using haircolor as your makeup.

To broaden or lift a forehead that is too small or too low The trick here is to use highlighting around the face only. Adding light around the forehead gives the illusion of "opening up" the whole area, or helping the forehead to appear broader.

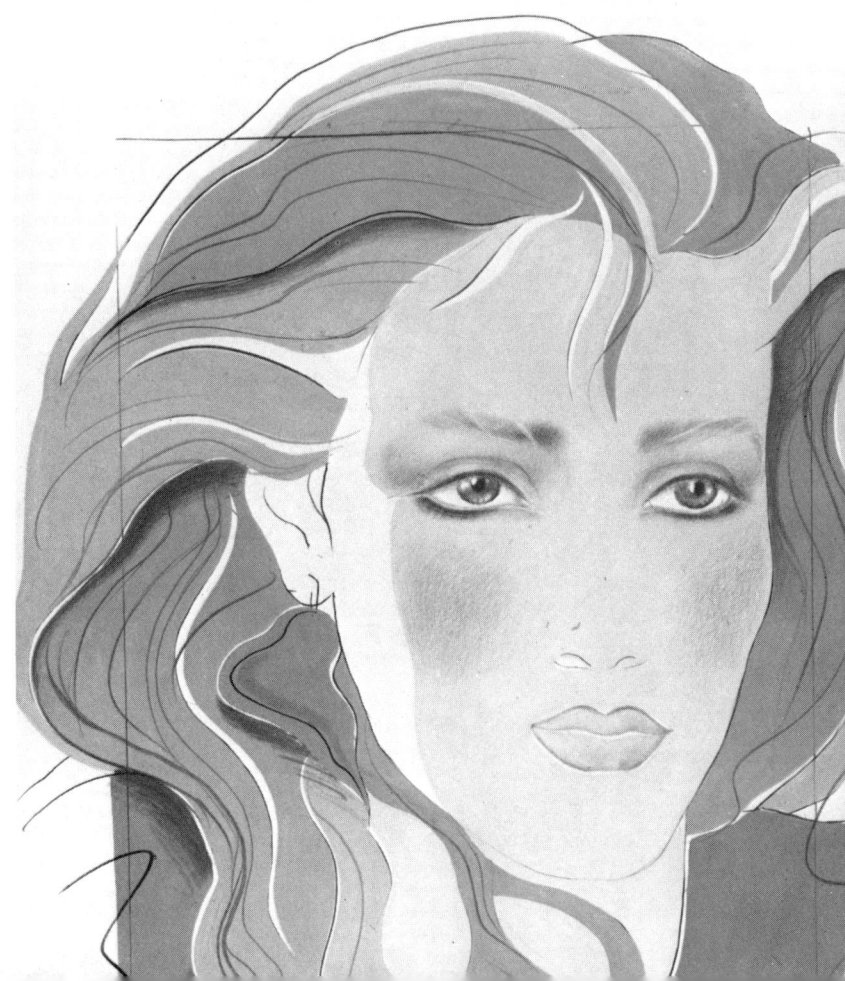

Uplifting droopy eyes To give droopy eyes an uplift, add a few bright highlights on the bangs or hair just above each eye. This will take away the "heavy" look from droopy or bedroom eyes and give the illusion of adding light and sparkle. While you're at it, consider lightening your eyebrows slightly if they are adding to the heaviness of the total eye area.

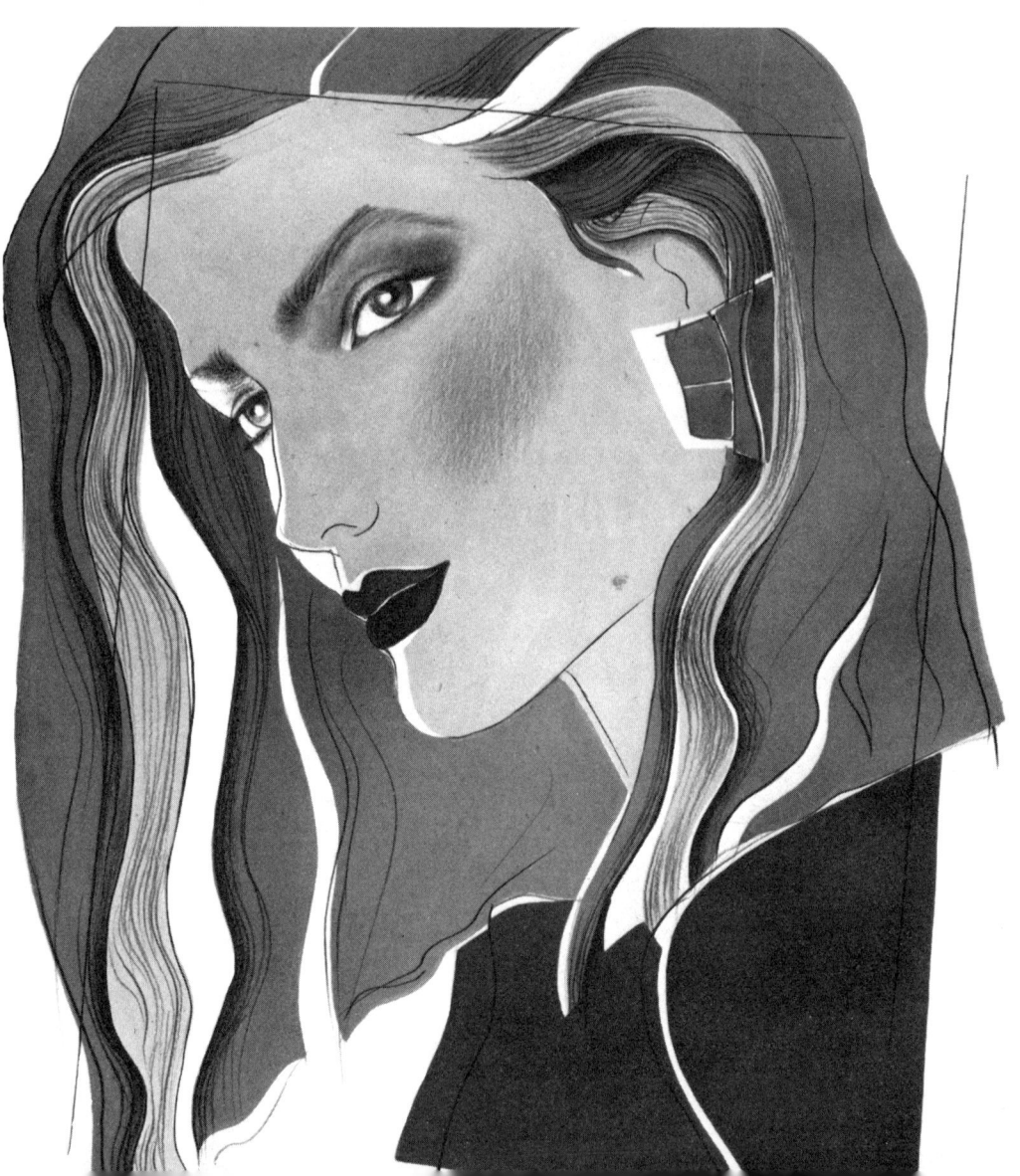

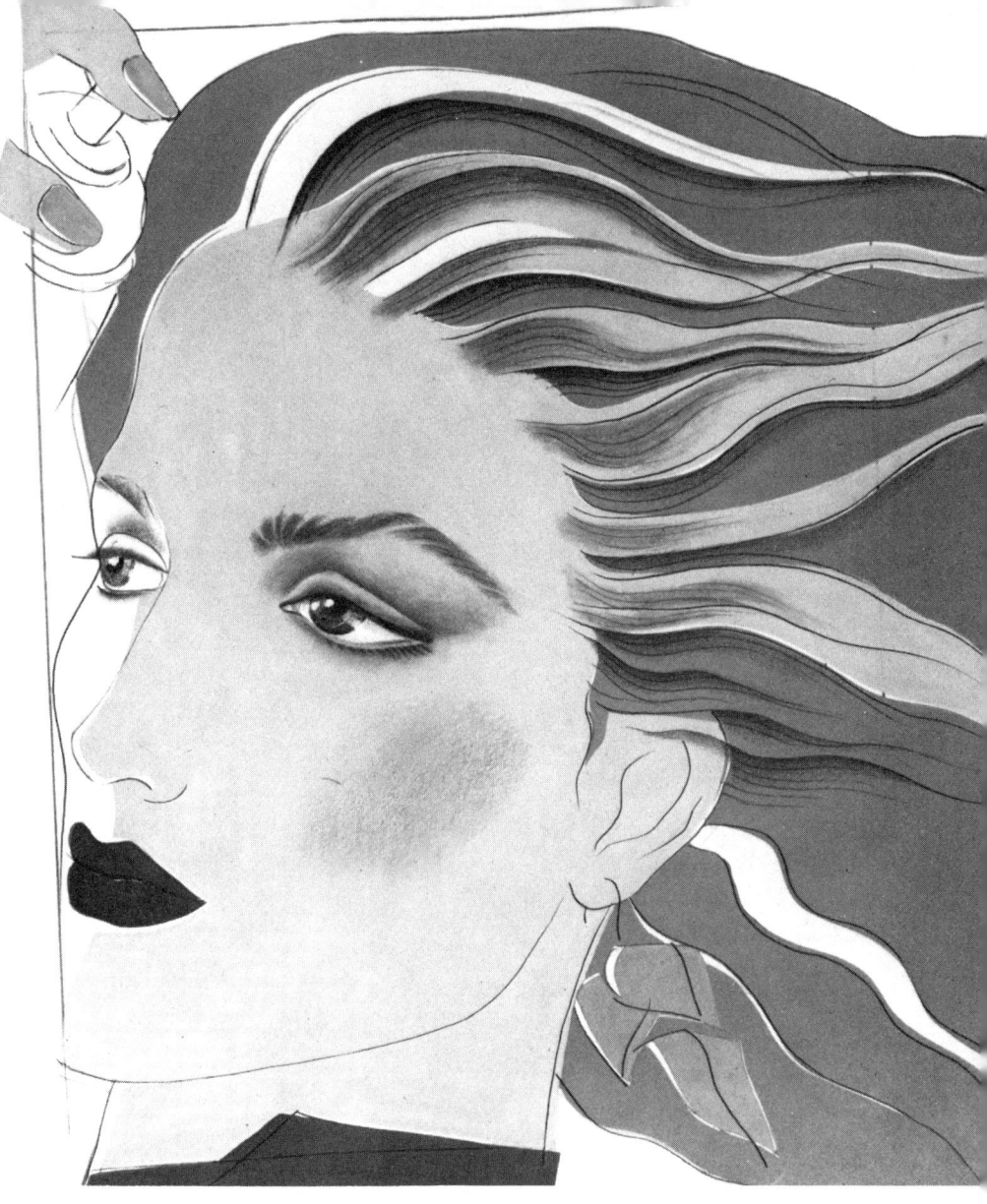

To narrow a wide, round face If the face is too wide or round, try a technique called lowlighting which is illustrated in chapter 5. As opposed to highlighting, which adds light tones, lowlighting creates deeper, warmer tones on selected strands of hair. For a round face, lowlights should be placed more heavily at the sides of the face and at the top of the head. These deeper tones, however subtle, will create the illusion of a longer, thinner look.

To widen a narrow, thin face   If the facial area is too narrow, concentrate some highlights just at the sides, adding only a few highlights at the top. This creates the illusion of a wider face.

To minimize a double chin   What we want to do is take away the attention from the double chin and lead the eye completely from this area. We achieve this by adding highlights exclusively in the top section of our hairstyle, because the eye always travels most quickly to the lightest part of the hair. To further minimize a double chin, hair should be cut to about chin-length (no shorter) and cut blunter so that all the weight of the cut and depth of the color are at the bottom, and all the light is at the top.

To minimize a large nose   To help soften the line of a large nose, eliminate any type of central hair part. Hair should, instead, be parted off the side to throw attention off the hard line of the nose. The bang section should be soft and fringy; highlighting this section will add to a light feeling around the forehead. This asymmetric feeling will keep a larger nose from being the center of attention.

Getting Familiar With Color Talk

It helps to review some of the most common terms used in haircoloring, the jargon, if you will. You'll see and hear these terms on packages, in beauty articles and in salons. Get familiar

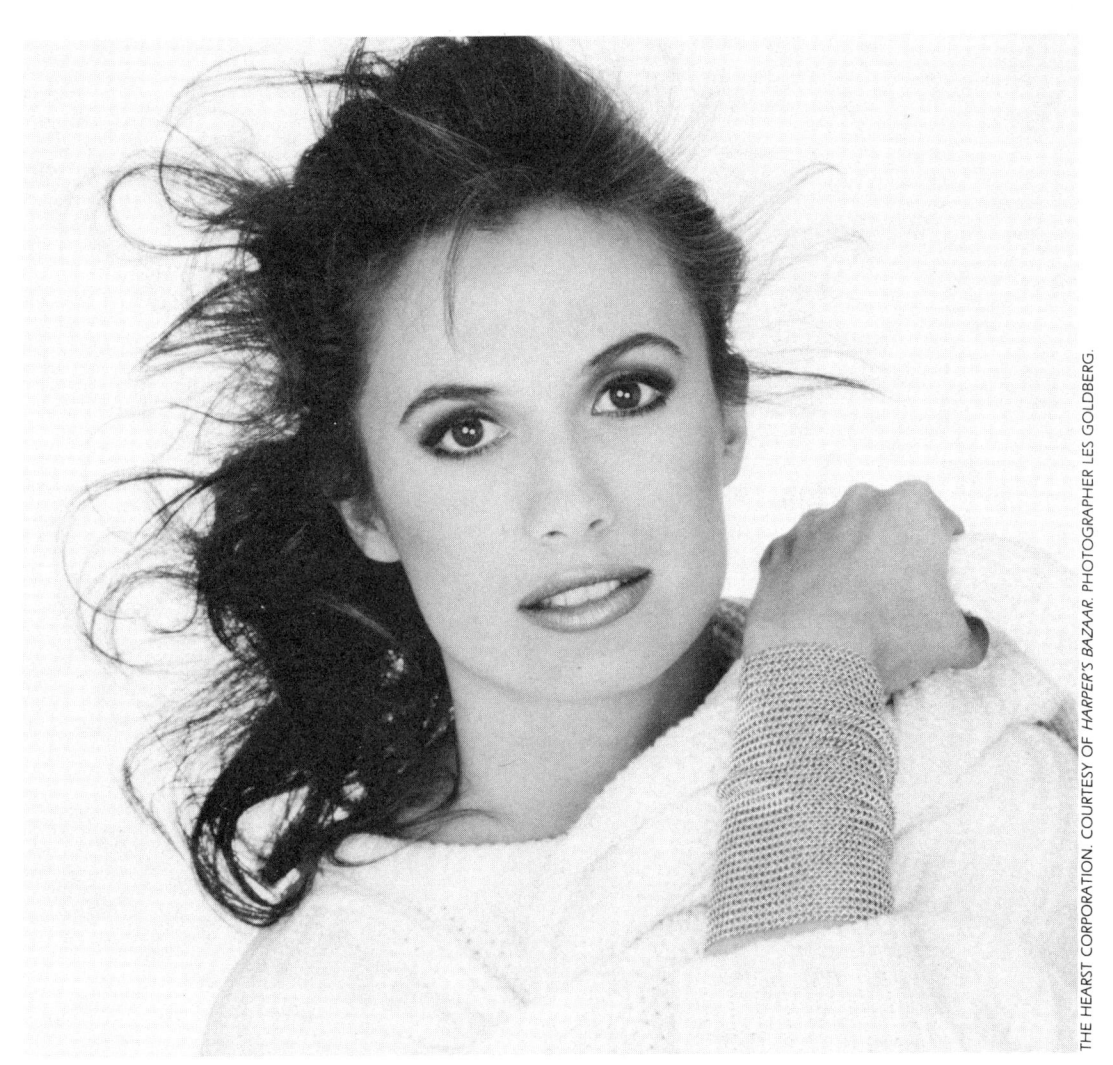

Beautiful Ana Alicia of "Falcon Crest" is the perfect example of what semipermanent haircolor can do for brown hair—add soft, natural, golden lights.

"I think of myself as a lively brunette," says Ana, who lives in California. "I feel my best when the sun lightens my hair and tans my skin. In the winter, my hair is darker and my skin very fair—it's a soft look that I also love."

Ana always looks beautiful to me, in any season. Her soft, rich haircolor is a big part of her fashion image.

with different aspects of haircolor; then the decision about what to use, when to use it and how will be much easier. Here they are. . . .

Temporary colors, also known as rinses, coat the outside of the hair shaft (the cuticle) with color which will wash out during the next shampoo. They don't contain peroxide so they cannot lighten your hair or actually change its natural color. They don't provide top coverage but they're fine for refreshing permanent color between touch-ups. I think they're great for first-time color users who want to try out or preview a color. They know that they can wash out the color right after their first experiment.

Semipermanent colors last from four to six shampoos and generally provide better coverage than temporary colors. Semipermanent colors also contain no peroxide. They are often prepared as foams and lotions. The lotions tend to last longer on the hair and the foams are easier to apply . . . take your pick. This type of coloring can enrich or deepen your natural hair color but cannot help lighten your hair. Semipermanent colors add brightness and help blend in gray.

Permanent color (tints) can actually change the hair's color by chemically altering the hair's structure to be either lighter or darker. Along with actually adding new color to the hair, permanent color mixtures lighten the hair to remove the natural pigment. As the name clearly states, the color imparted is "permanent." It will not wash out!

Highlighting is designed to warm up your hair with tones of red and/or sunny glints of blond. It is a wonderful way to bring so-called "drab" hair to life. Highlights are subtle, but permanent. They, too, won't wash out. They also need retouching

Permanent color adds long-lasting, rich tones.

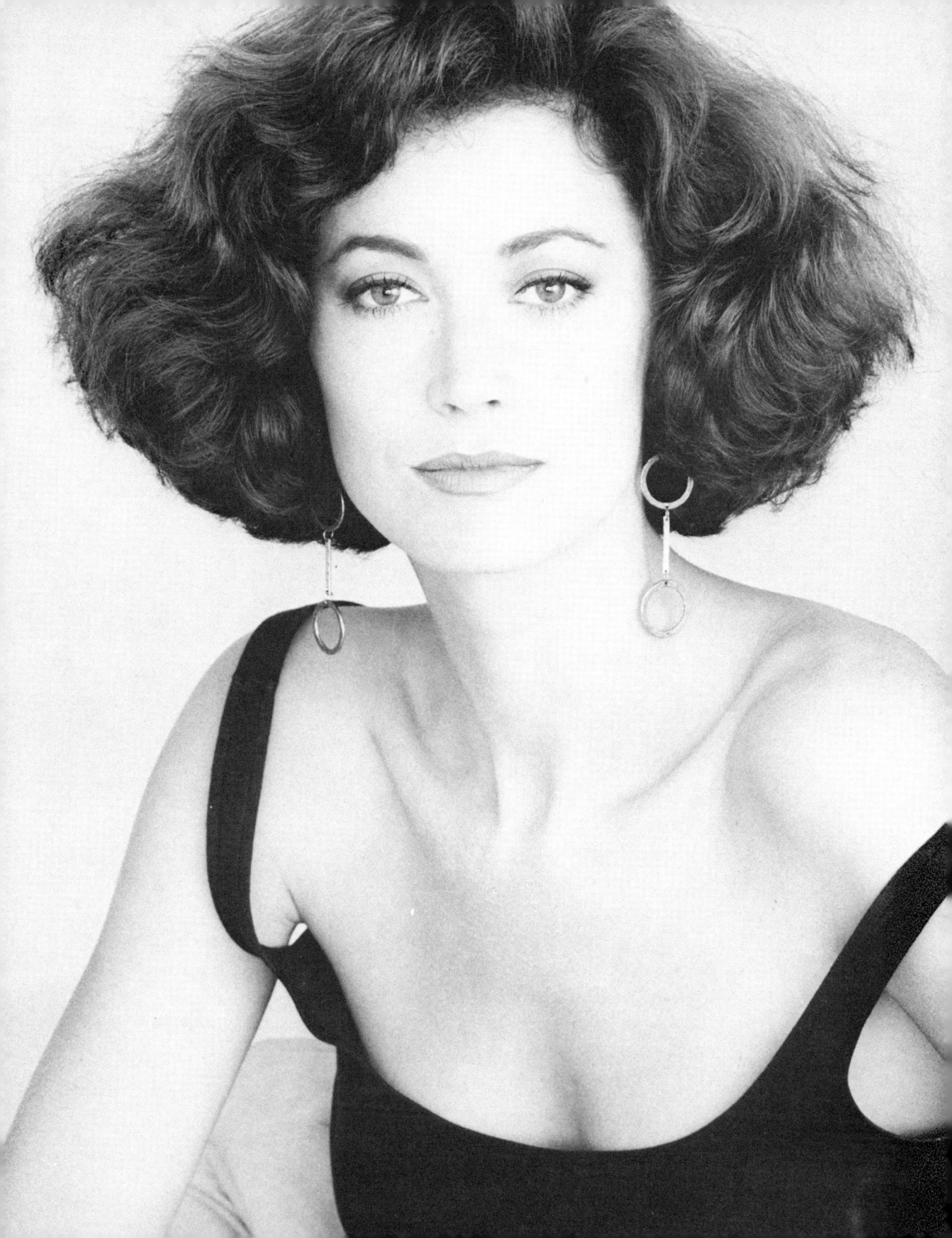

every three to six months depending on how heavily the hair is highlighted, the lightness of the color and how quickly the hair grows. Highlighting kits are easy to use. All you have to do is paint the lightener on the selected strands of hair.

Streaking is the same process as highlighting except that you create the illusion of blonde without a complete change in your natural haircolor by distributing the lighter strands all over the head. Streaking provides more color contrast and a more striking effect than highlighting. Touch-ups are not needed for three to four months at a time.

Two-step coloring is very straightforward. The first step actually lightens the hair shaft, removing the hair's natural color and preparing it to take on the shade we choose. Step two is the application of the color you want your hair to have (see *toning* below). Obviously, the color imparted is permanent.

Toning the hair refers to the second step of the two-step coloring process. Toners provide the final desired shade of color for your hair. They can also be used on their own to refresh a highlighting or to tone down the yellow of graying hair and the brassiness of some reds and blonds.

Oxidation, as it refers to hair color, is the "aging" or "curing" process of a new hair coloring. As a result of the chemical interaction of the oxygen in the air and the haircoloring ingredients, a new hair color comes to its truest and richest result only after a few days.

Retouching is the term used for coloring only the root area of the hair shaft, the quarter to half an inch of hair at the scalp that doesn't match the shade of the rest of the hair shaft. These roots, or "regrowth areas," appear about four to six weeks after the initial application of permanent haircolor. This is when retouching the roots is necessary with matching color. It's im-

Top model Roseanne Vela is the perfect example of the beauty of highlighting.

portant to remember that the closer you stay to your natural haircolor, the less the contrast between your roots and the rest of the hair shaft. *Note:* Touch-ups are easy and fast to do today. Roots used to be a negative word in haircoloring; now it simply means another maintenance step in our beauty regimen, like giving yourself a monthly deep-conditioning treatment or treating your skin to a great facial.

Turning Terms into Techniques

Now that you're familiar with the major terms used in haircoloring, take a look at the chart that follows. It will give you more information to add to your new and rapidly increasing knowledge of color.

Choosing the Right Color

If you've never colored your hair before, it's best to choose a color that is close to your own shade or slightly lighter. Lighter shades look better on most people; they are flattering to most skin tones.

For do-it-yourselfers, the haircoloring packages will give you an idea how various shades will look on your hair. However, the resulting color always depends upon your natural hair color; the only way you can really determine how it will look is to try it out. Follow the package directions for the strand test. (See pages 80–82).

Above all, your choice of haircolor definitely should take into consideration your natural complexion. A medium-blonde

Guide to Haircoloring Methods

	PERMANENT COLOR	SEMIPERMANENT COLOR	TWO-STEP COLOR	HIGHLIGHTING/ STREAKING
WHAT WILL IT DO?	Lighten or darken a few shades; make your own color prettier; cover gray.	Enhance your own hair color; cover gray; will not lighten.	Lighten dark hair to pale blond without red undertones.	Lighten selected strands of hair—as little or as much as you like.
HOW DOES IT WORK?	Shampoo in. Wait 20 minutes. Rinse or shampoo out, according to directions.	Apply. Wait 20–45 minutes. Rinse out.	Two Steps: First apply lightener for specified time. Shampoo out. Then apply toner. Shampoo out.	Apply lightener to selected hair strands. Follow directions for time and method.
HOW LONG WILL IT LAST?	Until the hair grows out; reapply once a month.	Through 4–5 shampoos; it's nonperoxide; wears away gradually.	Until the hair grows out; reapply once a month.	Until the hair grows out; apply to new hair strands 3–4 times a year.
HOW TO CHOOSE THE SHADE	Check the color chart on the package. Your own hair color will affect the color results.	Choose shades close to your own hair color.	Select any toner shade you like when you buy the lightener kit.	Key it to your present color.
SPECIAL TIPS	Provides greatest coverage of gray.	Lighter colors are generally more flattering.	Read toner instructions first to see how much to lighten your hair.	Start with a little highlighting—you can always do more if you want.

with very rosy skin, for example, would want to create subtle ash highlights to play up her skin tones and eye color. On the other hand, the same medium-blonde with pale, sallow skin should stay away from ash tones; they accent the sallow quality of the skin. Instead, she should choose light neutral blond highlights to enhance her total color image.

Find your natural haircolor and skin tones on the following chart, and you'll know the exact color to choose for a more beautiful you.

What happens if your haircolor doesn't turn out right? If you've gone to a salon, don't be afraid to tell your colorist. He wants to make you happy and has the ability to adjust your color immediately.

If you're a do-it-yourselfer and your color is darker than you

Hair Color Options

HAIRCOLOR		VERY PALE SKIN	PALE & ROSY SKIN	PALE & SALLOW SKIN	VERY ROSY SKIN	OLIVE SKIN
MEDIUM BLOND	Min.	Subtle Ash Highlights	Golden Blond Highlights	Light Neutral Blond Highlights	Subtle Ash Highlights	
	Max.	Lightest Baby Blond	Lightest Ash Blond	Light Neutral Blond	Medium Ash Blond	
DARK BLOND	Min.	Subtle Ash Highlights	Golden Blond Highlights	Light Neutral Blond Highlights	Subtle Ash Highlights	Delicate Golden Highlights
	Max.	Lightest Golden Blond	Lightest Ash Blond	Light Neutral Blond	Medium Ash Blond	Light Warm Blond
STRAWBERRY BLOND	Min.	Subtle Golden Highlights	Lighter Strawberry Highlights	Neutral Blond Highlights	Golden Highlights	
	Max.	Light Golden Blond	Lightest Ash Blond	Light Neutral Blond	Light Golden Blond	
BRIGHT RED	Min.	Subtle Reddish-Blond Highlights	Subtle Golden Highlights	Neutral Blond Highlights	Subtle Reddish-Blond Highlights	
	Max.	Light Strawberry Blond	Medium Ash Blond	Medium Neutral Blond	Medium Golden Blond	
AUBURN	Min.	Subtle Golden Highlights	Medium Reddish-Blond Highlights	Reddish-Blond Highlights	Coppery Highlights	Enriched Warm Highlights
	Max.	Light Honey Blond	Medium Ash Blond	Dark Golden Blond	Medium Golden Blond	Medium Reddish Blond
LIGHT BROWN	Min.	Subtle Golden Highlights	Light Golden Highlights	Reddish-Blond Highlights	Medium Ash Highlights	Warm Blond Highlights
	Max.	Light Honey Blond	Light Golden Blond	Medium Golden Blond	Medium Ash Blond	Light Blond
MEDIUM BROWN	Min.	Subtle Golden Highlights	Light Golden Highlights	Reddish-Blond Highlights	Medium Blond Highlights	Warm Blond Highlights
	Max.	Medium Blond	Light Golden Blond	Medium Golden Blond	Light Blond/Brown	Warm Blond Highlights
DARK BROWN/BLACK	Min.	Amber Highlights	Auburn Highlights	Light Brown Highlights	Light Ash Brown Highlights	Lightest Chestnut Highlights
	Max.	Light Warm Brown	Light Auburn	Light Brown	Light Ash Brown	Lightest Chestnut Brown

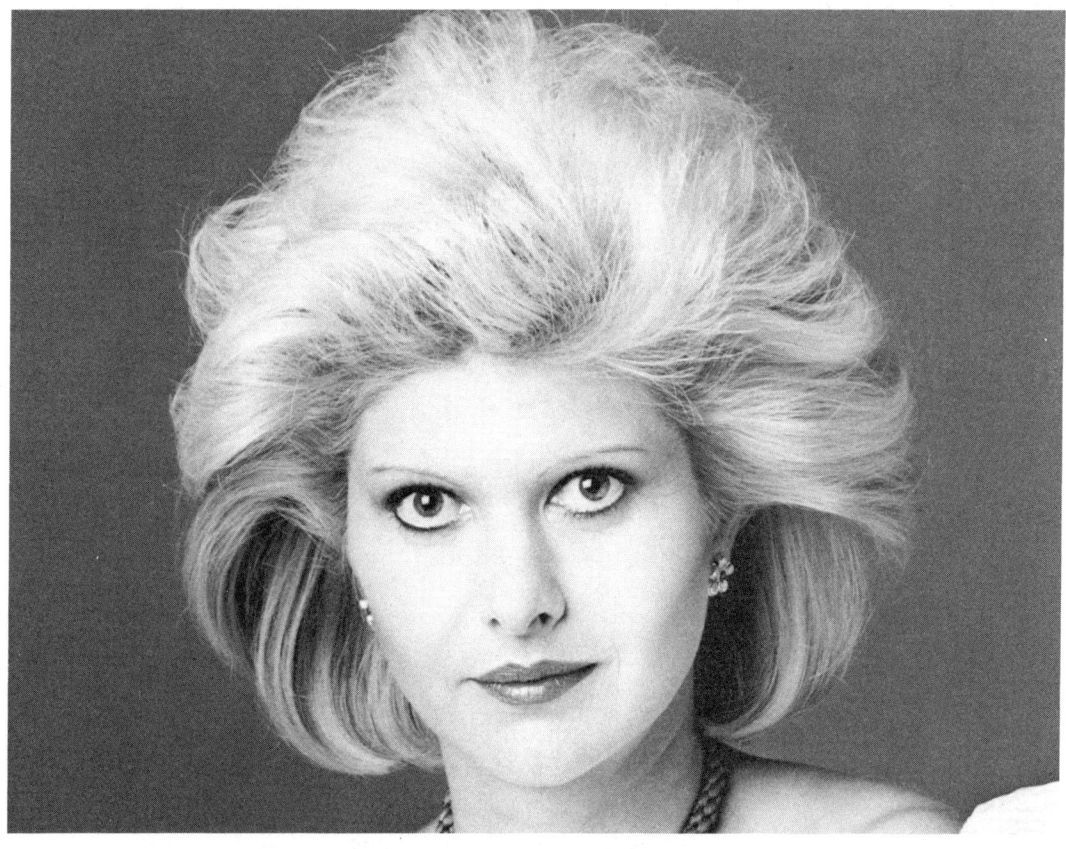

Ivana (Mrs. Donald) Trump is the perfect example of a person who has made the right color decision. One of those high-powered women who's bright and exuberant, she's noticed by all for her energy and beauty. A lot of this is because Mrs. Trump decided to become a blonde—the right shade of blond.

"I used to have very dark hair but I was always a blonde at heart," explains the lady who always fantasized about having "Brigitte Bardot blond." "When I decided to go blond, I loved it but quickly realized my blond was too white."

Mrs. Trump decided to see me for advice and subsequently became my client. Because her skin tone was an earthy olive shade, I made her white-blond hair a bit less severe by toning it down and making it more gentle and golden. I think Mrs. Trump will always be a blonde at heart, and now she has achieved the degree of blond that best suits her personality.

wanted, try shampooing once or twice right away to dilute the intensity or depth of a semipermanent or permanent color. If that doesn't work, shampoo two or three more times; this may be all you need to do to reach your desired shade.

Permanent shades that come out "way off" are also no cause for alarm. Simply call the "Haircolor Hotline" or Information Number listed on the instructions for the product used. There is a helpful haircolor consultant on the other end of the line twenty-four hours a day. She'll ask you some basic questions and usually recommend another shade that counteracts the color with which you were not satisfied. In some cases, she may suggest you see a salon haircolorist.

Salon vs. At-Home Haircoloring

There is a great variety of easy, creative haircolor techniques that you can do at home. However, only your professional salon haircolorist can give you the best results for certain techniques that require more skill, precision, and upkeep.

At-home products are easy to use and predictable even for the beginner as long as the directions are followed. You have excellent control and complete knowledge of exactly what shade your hair will turn out to be. This is because the manufacturers have taken out the "mystique" of haircolor. There is no magic involved; you are instructed what to do each and every step of the way.

As far as salon haircoloring, you may be the type of woman who feels more comfortable with a professional; you also may need an objective eye to recommend what's best for you. Other women merely enjoy the luxury of a salon itself.

Whether you're a high-powered businesswoman or a down-home, natural beauty, haircolor can fit into anyone's lifestyle.

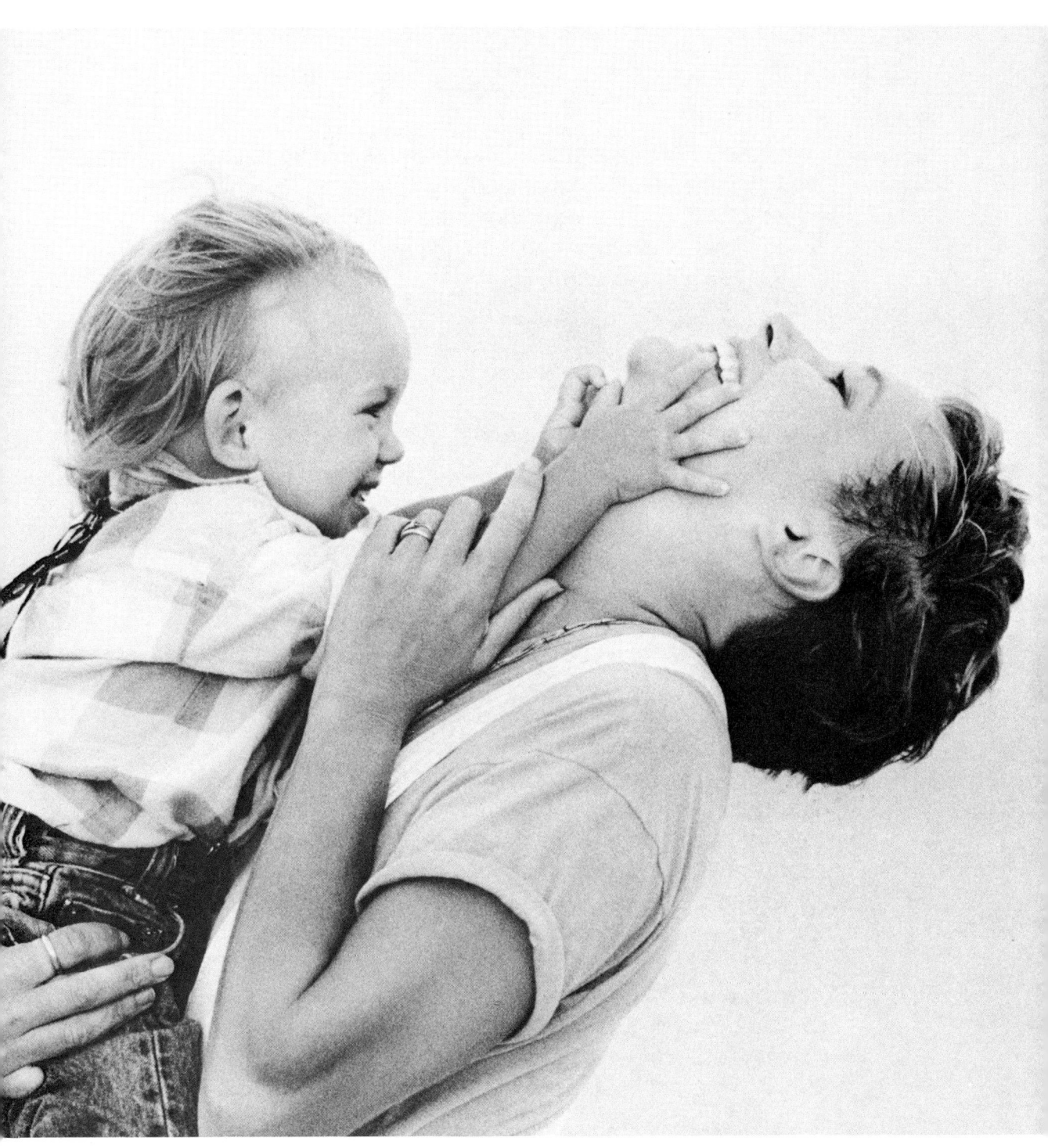

Whatever your choice, a salon haircolorist should be utilized by any woman thinking of coloring her hair. It makes good sense to consult with a professional about the direction you plan to take. Get his expert advice and creative approach before you begin. It can only help.

Take an Objective Look: Final Considerations

There are only a few more factors to consider as you make your haircoloring decisions. Each is a very important part of your total commitment to coloring your hair.

First, consider the cost. At-home color is obviously much less expensive than salon coloring, but think about what you want done and the worth of those final results. The cost depends literally on how often you color your hair. Do some costing out and you'll be sure to find a haircolor regimen within your own budget.

Consider the amount of time coloring your hair will take. Some techniques require more frequent touch-ups, like covering gray or keeping lightened hair from showing regrowth (especially if you have shorter hair). Highlighting, for example, needs to be done only three or four times a year. Other processes must be reapplied with every fourth to sixth shampoo.

If you go to a salon, your haircolorist will be able to explain how much time you should plan on spending in the salon and how often you must see him for a particular technique.

So there you have it—cost and time commitments that I'm sure you can work out within your own lifestyle. There is something beautiful for everyone. All you have to do is consider your many options and make your choice!

Chapter 3

Salon Haircoloring

When You Need a Professional

When you're thinking about coloring your hair, I recommend taking full advantage of the professional colorist at your salon. There are times when you absolutely should go to a professional, particularly when it's just plain smart to call upon his or her expertise.

To begin with, a pro has an objective eye. He or she will consider your type of hair, facial features, skin tones, lifestyle, personality, and overall image. As a result, the perfect haircolor can be created just for you. So if you look in the mirror and just don't know where to begin, get that expert, objective opinion.

A professional colorist also has a trained fashion awareness and artistic approach that has been developed over years of experience in the beauty business. He knows the latest trends, and can give you an exciting, contemporary haircolor effect—

something you may have seen only on those gorgeous models in the fashion magazines. If you want a total fashion image update, see your professional.

There are also special types of haircolor techniques that require precision, exact timing, total control, and even custom blending of colors that only a salon colorist is trained to do. Custom blending is mixing multiple colors to individualize your formula.

One of the techniques is foil highlighting, a highly refined concentration of highlights expertly woven throughout the hair. Selected strands of hair are placed gently in foils, covered with a lightening or color mixture, and then wrapped in the foil to let the coloring develop only where it's wanted. Placement of the foils and the total control of timing is vital here, and requires the watchful eye of the colorist.

Foil highlighting must be retouched with expert precision three to four times a year. Only the salon colorist knows how to touch up the regrowth areas so they blend with the rest of the hair shaft. He actually can match root to end, an extremely difficult technique.

There are several techniques involving permanent haircolor that I would suggest having done at the salon rather than at home. One of these occurs when you want a rather dramatic change in your color—like going from brunette to red or from red to blond; in other words, totally changing your "family" of haircolor. These changes are possible thanks to permanent color, but they usually require careful timing as well as the skilled eye of the colorist to bring you to the right degree of color within the desired range.

Another area of permanent color that's best left to the salon

To get the best results with two-step coloring, it's wise to see a professional.

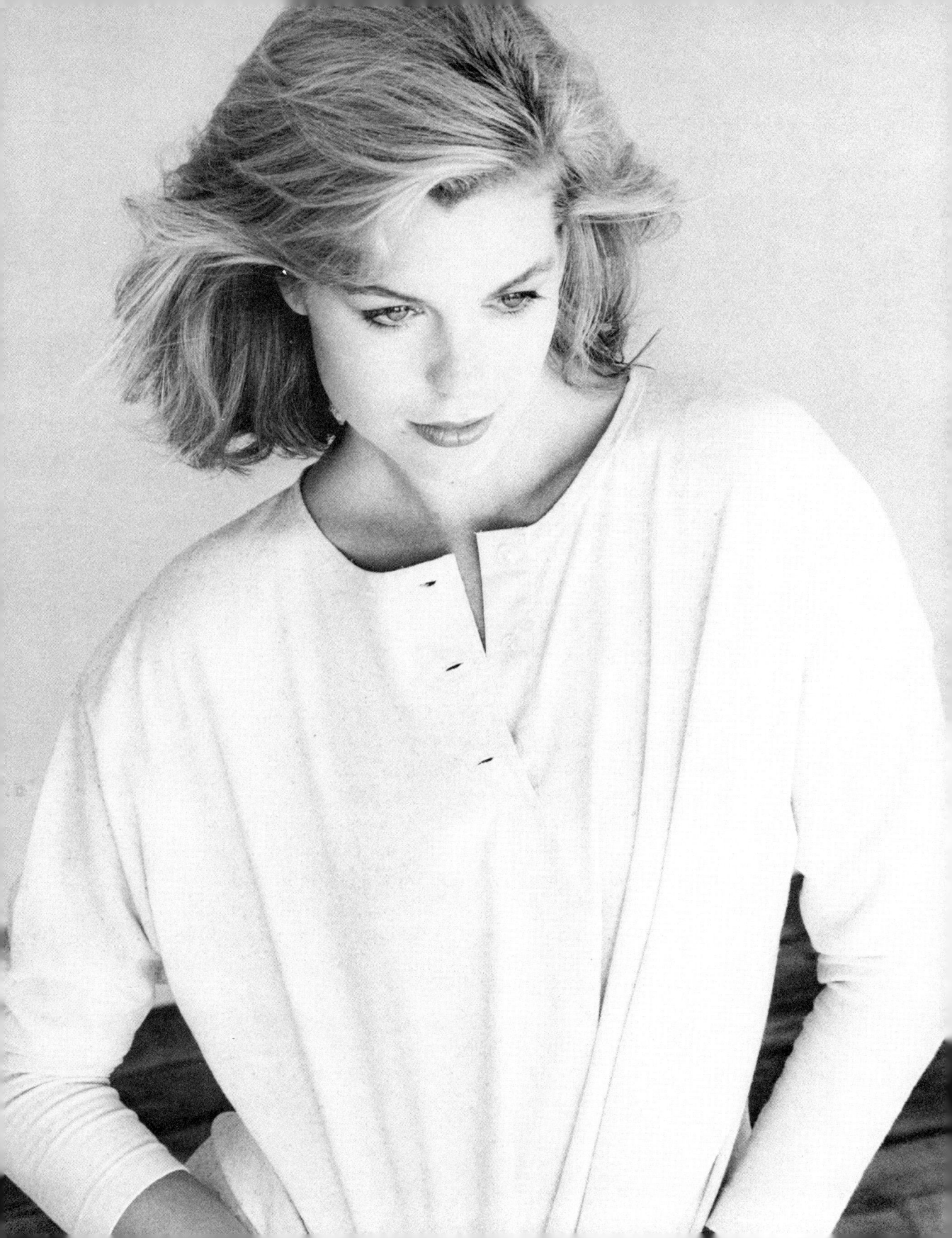

professional is two-step coloring which often means going much blonder than your natural color. Again, timing and total control of mixing and blending color is vital for successful results.

Corrective coloring is certainly an area that can only be handled by a pro. A woman who needs corrective measures—for example, if her haircolor is all wrong for her appearance or has somehow gone "beyond her control"—requires the fast advice and expertise of the salon colorist. What may seem an impossible situation to solve at home will be simple for the trained professional who knows exactly what steps to take for the right color adjustment.

How to Find the Right Colorist

A good way to begin the selection of a professional colorist is to get several recommendations from your friends or regular hairdresser. Then, make an appointment with each for a consultation so you can carefully assess whether the two of you agree on haircoloring. This consultation should be complimentary, or the fee should be applied toward your first color appointment. This process may sound time-consuming but most types of haircoloring are not like a dress you've decided you don't like—you can't slip out of them. You've got to wear it, so ask yourself the following questions.

1 Do you and the colorist agree about the look that's right for your hair? If you have to push your opinions at the person

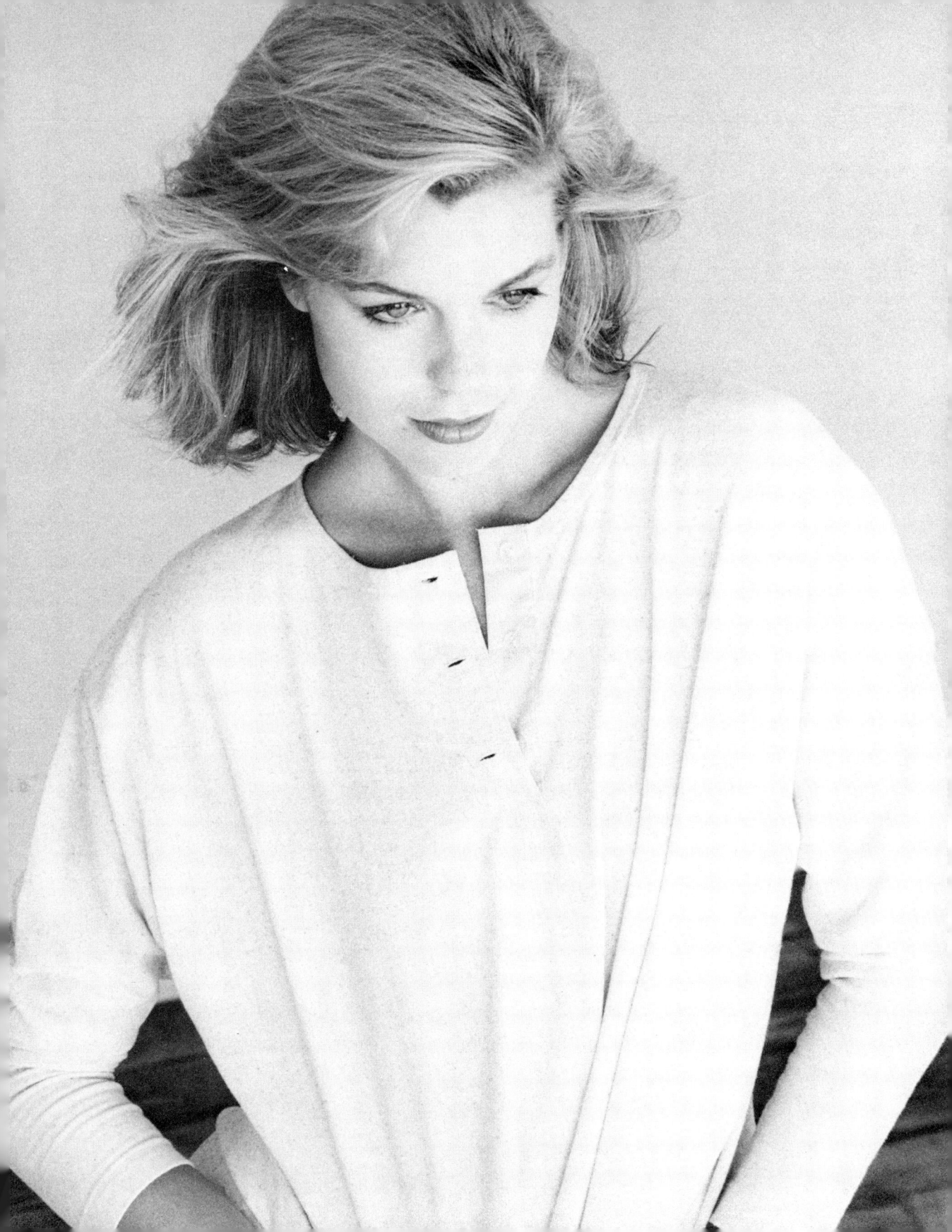

professional is two-step coloring which often means going much blonder than your natural color. Again, timing and total control of mixing and blending color is vital for successful results.

Corrective coloring is certainly an area that can only be handled by a pro. A woman who needs corrective measures—for example, if her haircolor is all wrong for her appearance or has somehow gone "beyond her control"—requires the fast advice and expertise of the salon colorist. What may seem an impossible situation to solve at home will be simple for the trained professional who knows exactly what steps to take for the right color adjustment.

How to Find the Right Colorist

A good way to begin the selection of a professional colorist is to get several recommendations from your friends or regular hairdresser. Then, make an appointment with each for a consultation so you can carefully assess whether the two of you agree on haircoloring. This consultation should be complimentary, or the fee should be applied toward your first color appointment. This process may sound time-consuming but most types of haircoloring are not like a dress you've decided you don't like—you can't slip out of them. You've got to wear it, so ask yourself the following questions.

1 Do you and the colorist agree about the look that's right for your hair? If you have to push your opinions at the person

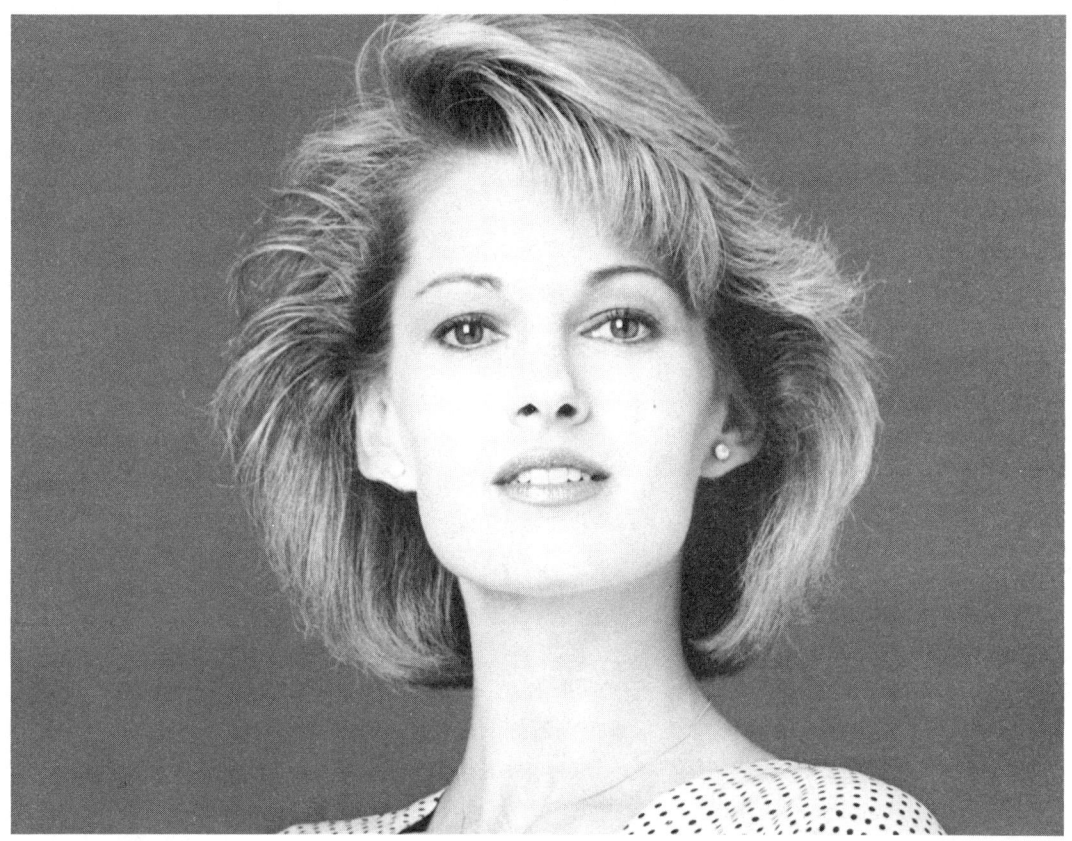

I think Cyndy Garvey is an appropriate example of how a woman really benefits from choosing the right salon colorist. Though she is a model, an actress, and talented cohost of talk shows, she has a lot in common with millions of women who need a fashion update of some sort and trust a professional to work with them.

"When I heard Louis tell the other clients around me that he wanted to create totally natural-looking color for them, I knew he was the colorist for me—right to the point and a no-fuss type of professional. He brought me from an "ash" California blonde to a natural, believable New York blonde all because he knew how to bring out my real personality."

I use a special foil highlighting technique on Cyndy's hair that creates allover highlights that continue to look better and better when she's under the sun—which is a lot in her sporty lifestyle.

during a consultation, they may be totally disregarded when his actual work begins.

2   How do you feel about the work he or she does? Is the caliber up to your standards? Other customers are usually pretty good indications of what the salon and the colorist turn out. If you love what you see on clients, you'll love what the colorist can do for you.

3   Is the colorist pleasant and willing to take time out to discuss your needs? This is very important, you want to be treated as an individual, not like an assembly line object or another head of hair.

4   Are you willing to pay the prices asked and spend the maintenance time suggested? If your schedule and budget are too tight for a long coloring process and frequent touch-ups, you'll want to look for a salon or method that won't tie you down.

5   Are the salon hours for haircoloring compatible with your own schedule or lifestyle? It's important that your colorist can accommodate your schedule, but also consider his or hers. Don't call and beg for an appointment at the last minute because you waited to get your color done. He'll work very well with you if the salon has adequate advance notice when booking appointments. A tip—don't forget to ask how long you should plan on being at the salon and adjust your time accordingly. Some haircolor procedures take longer than others.

A Fashion Show of Haircolor

How can you make beautiful women even more beautiful? With haircolor, of course. These top cover girls, modeling the newest haircolor fashion trends, represent how modern haircolor can make the difference between looking good and looking fabulous.

These colorful pages offer a variety of exciting haircolor options. The choice is yours.

Roseanne Vela

The first special effect, called chameleon colors, is a rich blend of contrasting highlights.

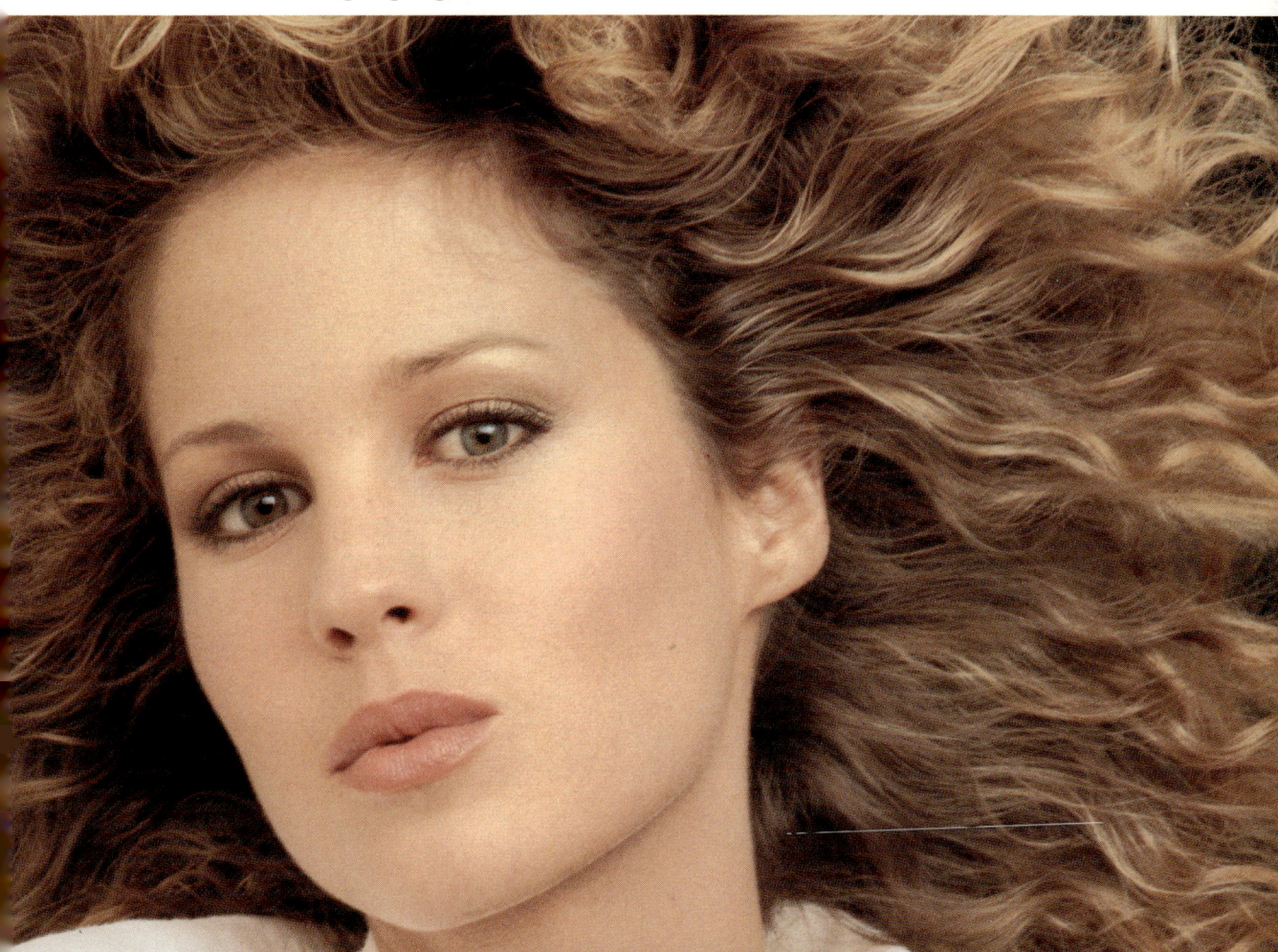

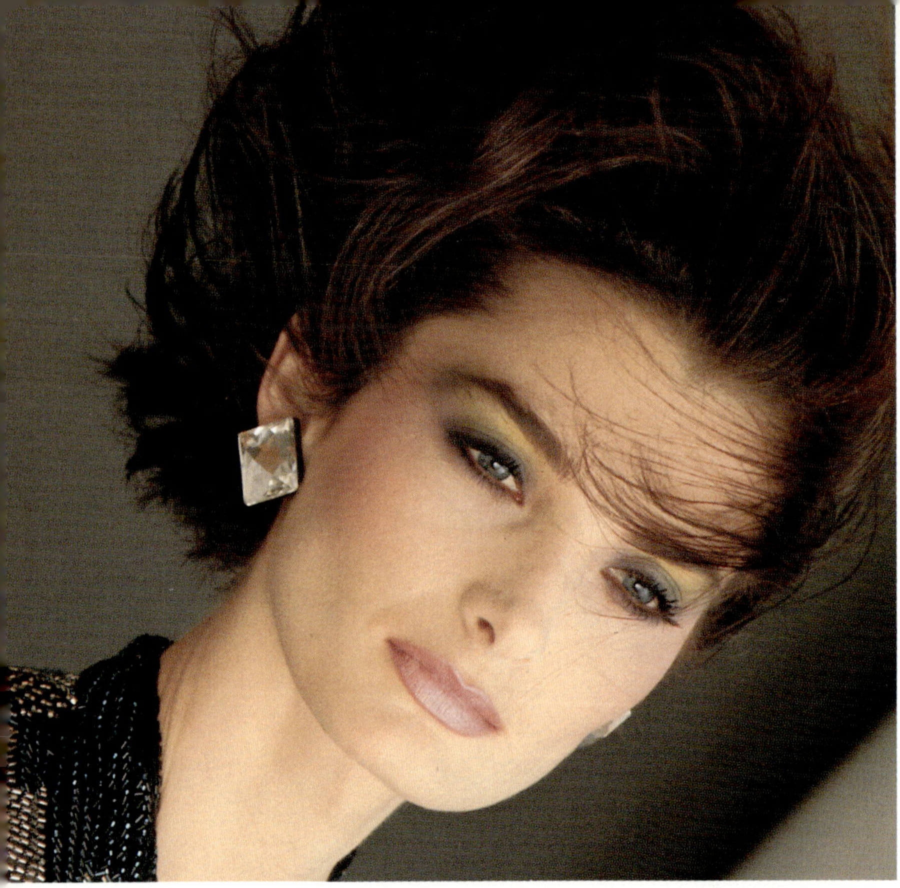

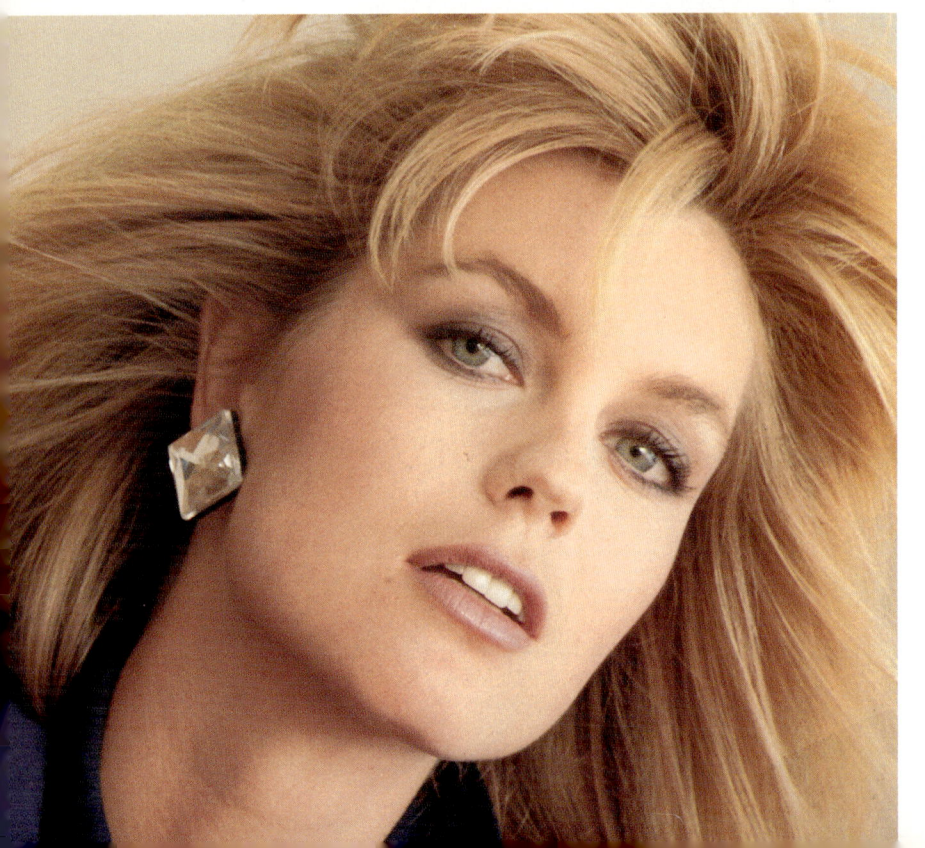

Margaret Donohoe

You don't have to think of neon when it comes to nite-glittering. It can look soft and subtle under the night lights.

Donna Sexton

Silhouettes are highlights that accent the shape of your hairstyle.

Tara Shannon

Glazing creates a highly polished sheen while bringing out rich vibrant color.

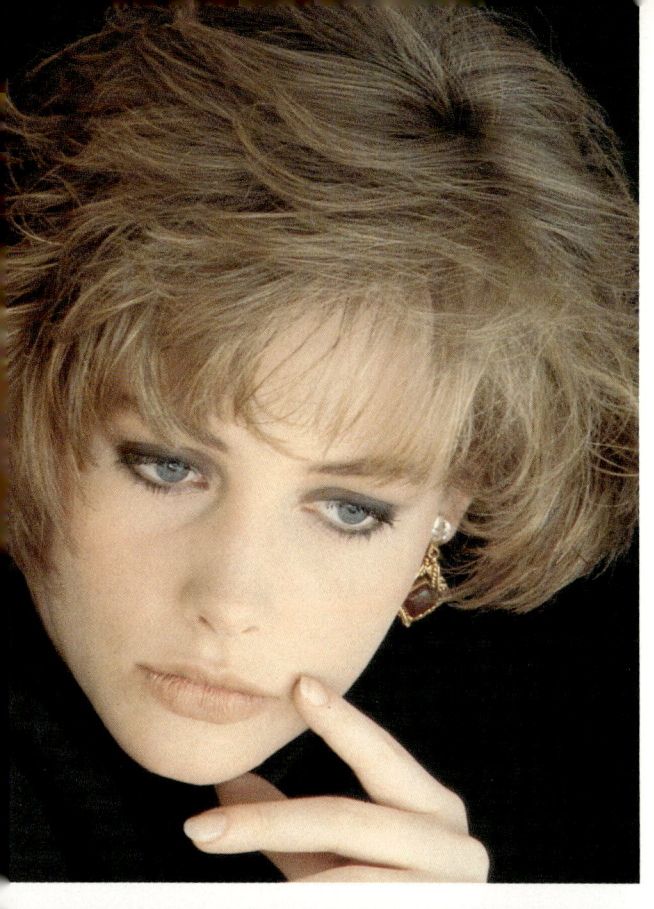

Lauren Helm

Another fashion technique is "illusions," a way to minimize facial flaws or simply to throw light around the face.

Ty Hendrick

Brush-on blushers can be used to add color accent at the temples and on top of the hair.

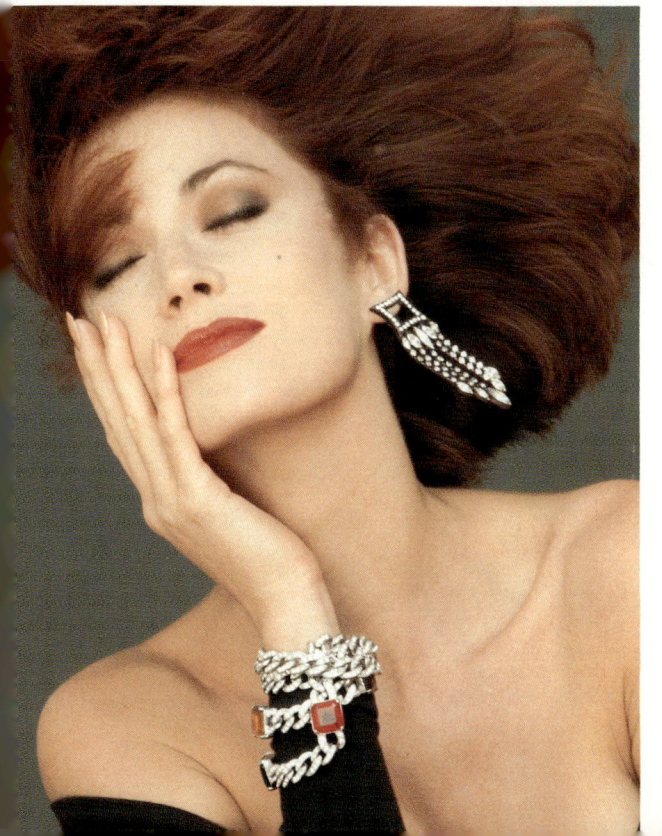

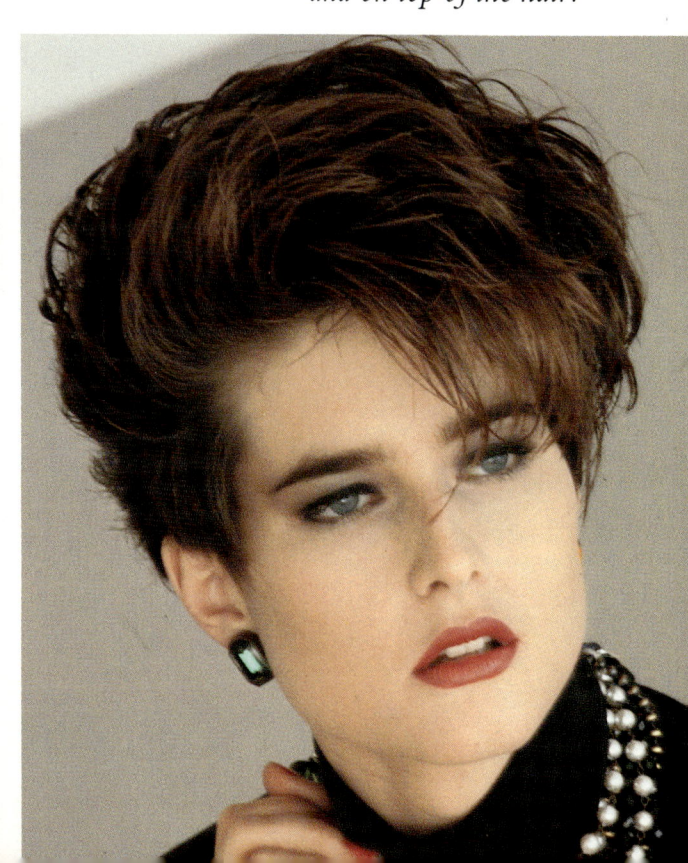

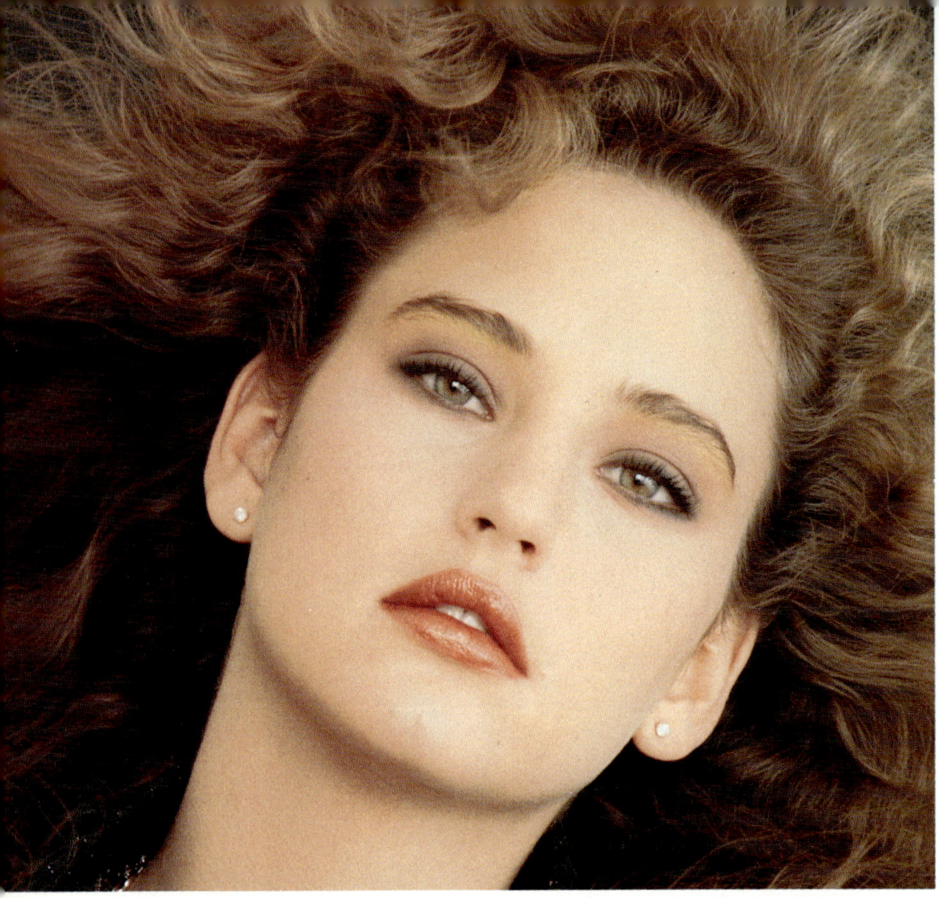

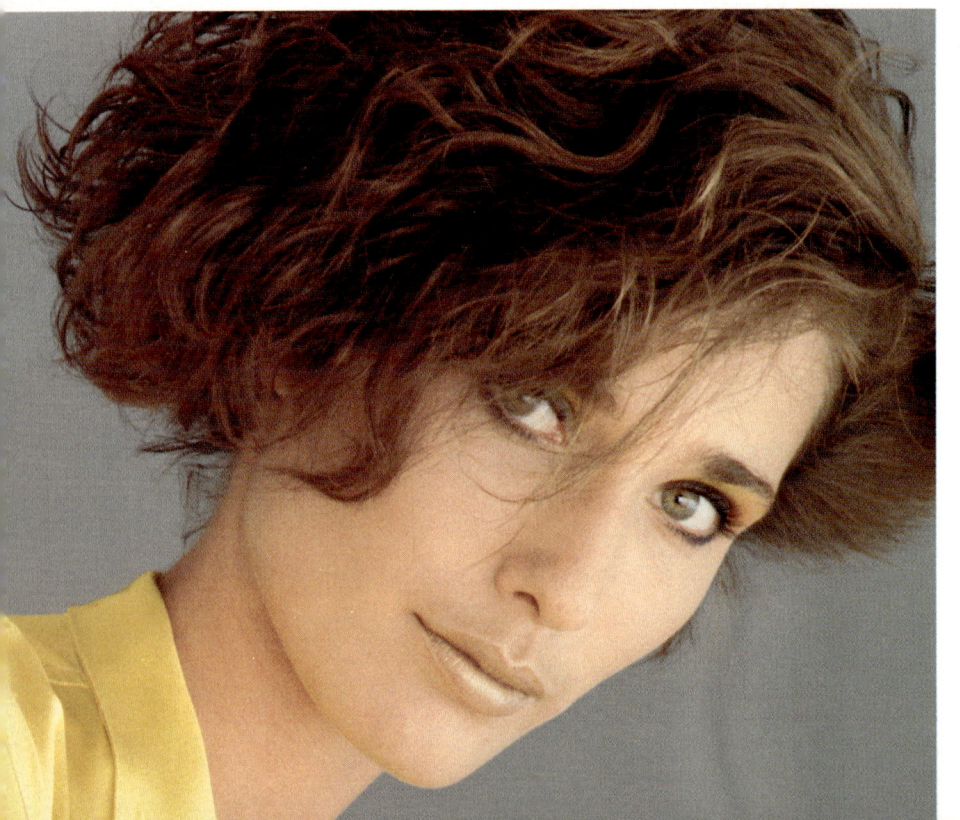

Jill Goodacre

Tie-dyeing adds soft waves of color to long hair.

Jen Yarrow

Color blocking accents a shorter cut by coloring specific sections of the hair.

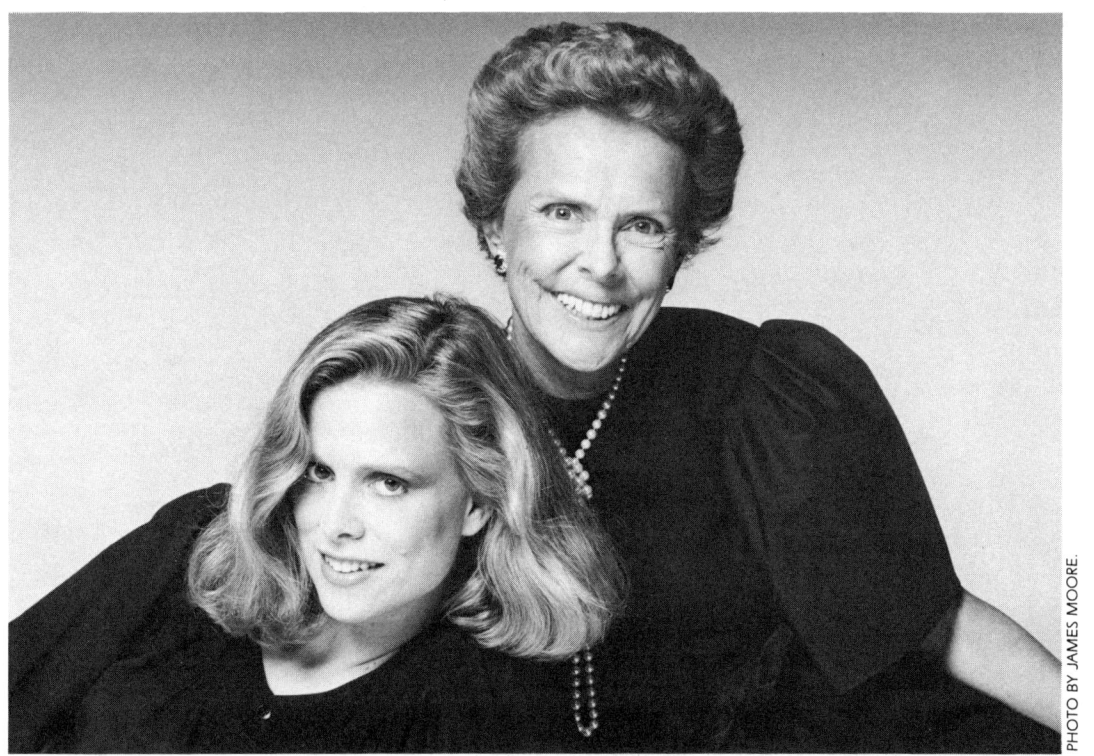

Owner of the world-renowned Ford Model Agency based in New York, Eileen Ford is definitely part of the cross-over clientele generation. So is her daughter Lacey. They truly are women of the eighties and, I believe, way ahead of their time in the fashion and beauty business.

Both women are clients who come to see me as regularly as their hectic schedules permit. They travel all around the world making appearances, researching trends, and seeking out the most beautiful girls in the world as prospective Ford models. Obviously, it's important for their haircolor to look its best at all times.

I would describe Mrs. Ford's haircolor as dark blond with highlights. Lacey's hair is foil-highlighted. To keep their colors looking fresh and alive while they are traveling, I give each her own personal color formula or "prescription" to apply herself or give to a salon in any part of the world.

This is a good example of how anyone can utilize the talents of her haircolor professional.

The Cross-Over Clientele Generation

A new phenomenon has occurred—I call it the cross-over clientele generation. These are women who now get their basic color work, like extensive highlighting, done at a salon about three to four times a year, while refreshing or touching up their color at home between salon visits. This is definitely a growing trend; women no longer have to choose "either/or." Instead they can have the best of both worlds of haircolor—at the salon and at home.

As I mentioned previously, every woman coloring her hair at home should also check with her salon once in a while, just to see if the colorist recommends any changes or ways to update her haircoloring. An expert has the ability to view clients objectively and perceive quickly the best changes for their overall images and modern appearances.

It is important to do something new with our haircolor on a regular basis, even if it's just a subtle change here and there. Our colorist can keep us on top of fashion changes, and keep our haircolor personality from looking dated.

A big part of the cross-over clientele generation is the woman who travels but also prefers custom-blended colors. She needs good basic semipermanent coloring done at the salon but doesn't have the time to return for touch-ups as regularly as she would like. I give many of these clients the formulas they will need to refresh or touch up their color until the next time I see them. This sharing of haircolor "recipes" keeps their color looking terrific wherever they go.

Clients who work long and demanding hours also need some at-home help after I do their basic coloring at the salon.

For those with basic highlighting, I recommend a semipermanent shade to refresh the color over the following few months. I even custom-blend a formula that can last all summer.

I find that the more at-home help I give my salon clients the more satisfied they are with me and their haircolor. I think it's the colorist's helpful and educational approach that keeps his clients coming back over the years.

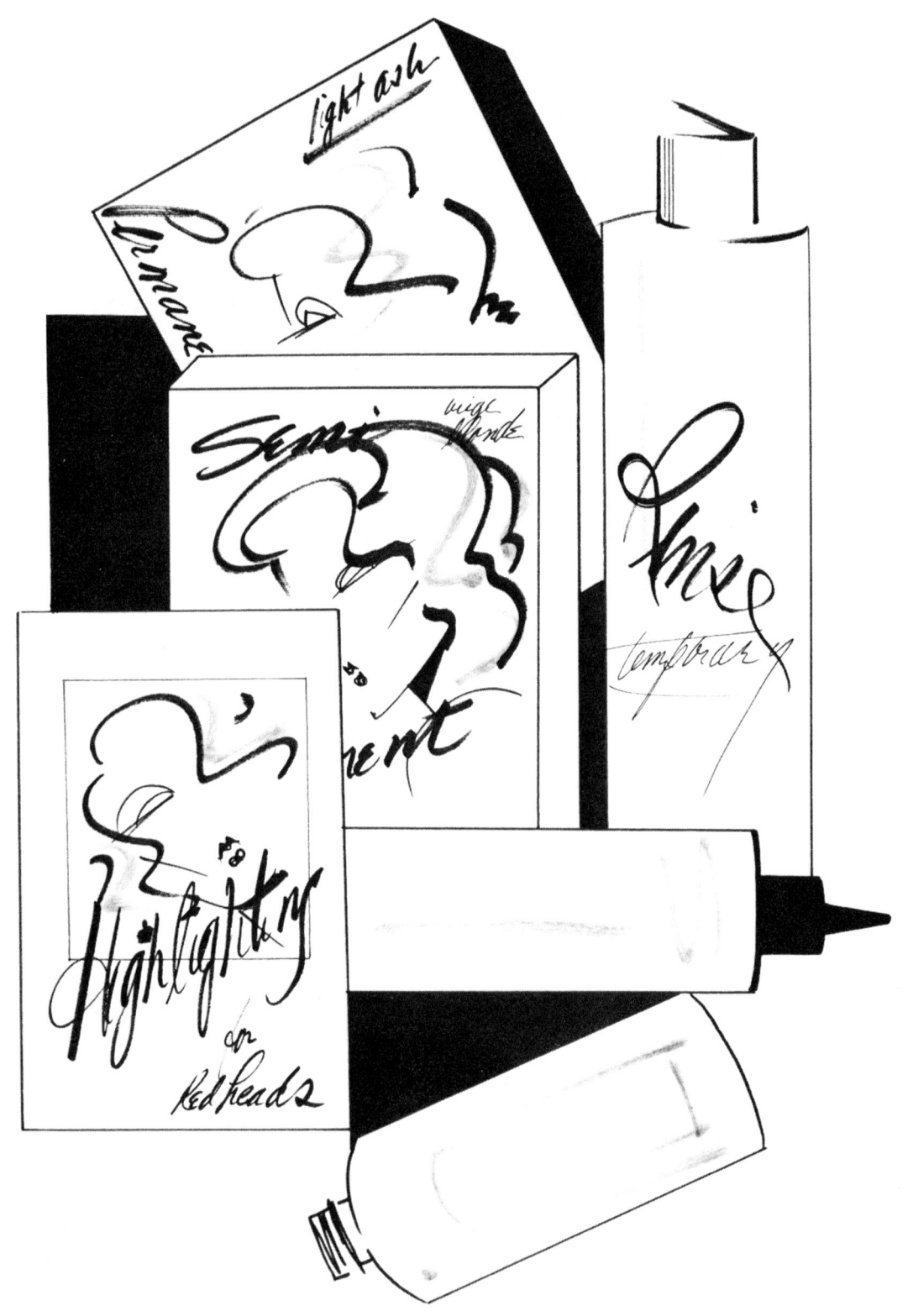

Chapter 4

The Wonderful World of At-Home Haircoloring: The Basics

Determining the Right Type of Product

One of the keys to determining the right at-home product is to pinpoint the length of time the color will last. This information, printed on every package of haircoloring, will specify whether the product is temporary, semipermanent, or permanent.

Unfortunately, each box is not marked according to these simple, clear categories of color. You will need to read the product description to determine this yourself; it's certainly worth taking the time to do so. You will find, however, that each category is grouped separately on the shelves—all temporary rinses are placed in one section, semipermanent colorings in another, and so on.

If you are at all confused about which product to buy, ask the salesperson in charge of the department. She or he is often called a retail cosmetician and has had some basic haircolor sales training from a haircolor manufacturer.

Now, let's review these major categories of haircolor again. This way, you'll really feel like an educated consumer.

TEMPORARY COLOR

Temporary color can be described best as a haircolor rinse that has a variety of uses. However, it will wash out with your next shampoo. This is because it only coats the hair shaft; it does not penetrate it or alter the natural color in any way.

Temporary color is particularly advantageous for the beginner who wants to try on or get a feeling for a new color without any lasting effects. Chances are, she'll like the results and quickly graduate to a semipermanent or permanent color.

Temporary colors are terrific for enhancing your own shade or creating a mood for a special occasion. Today, these types of colors range from the completely natural-looking to bright, dayglow effects. You can apply them all over or to special areas as in tie-dyeing.

Perhaps the most common use of temporary colors today is to tone down any brassiness in lightened hair. They are also used to refresh fading highlighted or streaked hair between basic applications, and to add some sparkle to dulling gray hair.

Remember that some temporary colors must be rinsed out when first applied; others should be left in to dry. They come in a variety of forms; I believe that the Roux rinses (like White Minx) in large plastic containers probably sell best because they are easy and fast to use.

Temporary color can also be found in shampoos for redheads or blondes. This is a good way to pick up some lights in your hair, but expect only a minimal change. Clairol's Shimmer Lights is a thicker, creamier shampoo that is especially good for refreshing blondes and toning down that yellow quality taken on by graying hair.

Finally, you can add some subtle highlights while styling your hair with the newest "mousse" styling foams on the market (these are basically styling aids with the added plus of temporary color built into them). Select the mousse specifically marked with your haircolor on the bottle: strawberry foams for redheads, lemon foams for blondes, and chocolate mousses for brunettes. Your own natural highlights will be picked up a bit and you'll have some fun in the process.

Temporary products undoubtedly are no-fuss haircolors. There's nothing to mix, and no patch or strand test needs to be done.

SEMIPERMANENT COLORS

These are my favorite. Semipermanent colors have a wonderful, rich, translucent quality that allow the natural nuances of your own haircolor to shine through. I think they are a beginner's best friend because they create a lovely soft color that's immediately apparent. The first-time user will have instant, visual proof that something wonderful has been done to her hair and total image.

Unlike temporary colors, semipermanents are more penetrating and last about four to six shampoos. They also require a patch and strand test before each application. Like temporary colors, they contain no peroxide and quietly fade away until your next overall application. There are no roots or regrowth area to touch up. You just shampoo—or foam—it in and watch your haircolor come alive.

Here's a visual example: Think of drawing a red crayon over a dark brown background. This red will become a deep reddish-brown rather than a true red. This is similar to how semipermanent color shows against darker hair. On light base shades, a dark semipermanent will darken the entire hair. Light shades on a light base really will not create any distinct difference. Regardless of the base shade, semipermanent colors do provide substantial coverage of gray, but please note that *permanent* colors are your best bet for *lasting* effects and total coverage.

Semipermanent colors come in either a lotion or a foam. The lotions coat the hair very well and are especially good for women who have long hair; the foams appear a bit easier to apply at home. Neither version is difficult to use, however.

Here are some tips for selecting a semipermanent shade:

1   When you simply want to cover gray and match your natural haircolor, choose a shade or two lighter than your own. This will be very flattering and close enough to your basic color. Watch your stray grays turn into soft highlights that blend with the rest of your color. This is what I call changing a defect into an asset.

2   If you want to enhance your own color, or add a bit of brightness or more vibrance, choose a shade that's slightly lighter, not darker, than your own. The results will be beautiful lights in your hair that really sparkle.

3 If your hair comes out too dark after semipermanent application, just shampoo to dilute the intensity of the color. If it's still too dark, continue shampooing until you reach the satisfactory color.

Given its easy-to-use, lovely-to-look-at qualities, I consider semipermanent coloring "minimum maintenance for maximum haircoloring effects."

PERMANENT COLOR

Permanent haircolor products have the ability to make the most dramatic changes. They are a one-step peroxide haircoloring that imparts more lasting color to just about any degree we wish. They can even lighten hair up to twelve shades or more as well as dramatically darken hair.

With natural-looking modern haircolor, however, we really don't need to utilize the full power and strength of the permanent colors. I always recommend not straying too far from your natural color as a general rule of thumb.

I believe that the real benefits of permanent color are to provide lasting true color (four to five weeks between touch-ups), give complete and lasting coverage of gray which is the most difficult hair to cover because it's porous, and to condition and improve the texture of the hair.

If you change the color of your hair significantly, you will have regrowth which requires regular touch-ups to keep the hair evenly colored from root to end. But this process has been made very easy for at-home use because haircolor mixtures have been made thicker for better control and ease of application—you can color only the root area with no overlapping onto the rest of the hair shaft.

One form of permanent haircoloring that I will not explore beyond this point is two-step coloring, also known as double-process color. This technique usually applies to women with darker hair who want to go much lighter. To achieve this dramatic change, the hair must be lightened dramatically to take away its natural dark pigment. Because this stage of blondness is usually too yellow to be worn as is, it's necessary to add a toner or a much warmer, usually blond, shade to bring hair to the desired color.

Frankly, I rarely recommend changing your color quite so dramatically, especially at home. I prefer to build up the natural color base of the hair rather than try to minimize or negate it in any way.

However, I do love toners when used by themselves. Categorized as a semipermanent type of color, they are wonderful for refreshing a highlighting or streaking, or toning down yellow in graying hair. They are also great for minimizing the brassiness in blonds and reds. Many of the contemporary shades of toners like a "true golden blond" or a "strawberry blond" add a certain warmth and richness to blondes that is outstanding. Like all other haircolor products, each toner box will tell you the color result to expect on your own shade of hair.

There are several types of permanent color products to choose from today. Nonammonia types like Clairesse have more appealing fragrance and create soft nuances in the hair yet they possess less lightening strength. Creme formulas create wonderful shine as well as color. Permanent colors also come in shampoo-in lotions and gels for excellent coverage and control.

All these products give you the same color results—the type you choose is a matter of personal preference. I usually recommend lotion forms of color if your hair is longer. Lotions distribute more evenly over lots of hair. Gels are terrific for shorter hair and are the easiest "no-fuss" permanent color on the market.

HIGHLIGHTING

Highlighting is the most popular form of haircolor. Because it is so easy to do and looks so natural, highlighting brought haircolor to the forefront of fashion. It was the one technique that was accepted immediately by women of all ages and lifestyles.

Highlighting is really a clever way to duplicate and play up what Mother Nature already gave us—beautiful light and dark tones throughout our hair. This technique can "warm up" your hair with fine coppery highlights or add shining glints of blond like the sun gives you.

If your hair tends to be drab, highlighting is an ideal way to brighten it. Highlights can be very subtle and should consist of very fine strands of hair to create the proper effect.

Highlighting is considered a permanent form of color because strands will simply remain lightened until they grow out or you cut them off. Plan to refresh or touch up highlights about three to four times a year.

I think the easiest highlighting kits for beginners are Clairol's Hair Painting kit and Clairol's Quiet Touch kit; just pick the kit geared to your natural base shade.

LOWLIGHTING

With the advent of modern haircolor, highlighting found a new friend called lowlighting. Instead of lightening selected strands, you *add color* to strands that is deeper and warmer than your natural color. This creates a beautiful tone-on-tone effect, and results in contrasts in the hair that look very natural.

There are no lowlighting kits, per se, on the market. The creative color choice is up to you—choose a shade in the semipermanent category for a deeper contrast to your own color and simply brush onto selected strands. Permanent color choices will simply last longer.

STREAKING

This is a popular at-home haircoloring technique that distributes a lot of very fine light strands all over the head, giving hair the illusion of being more blond than it actually is.

Streaking (formerly known as frosting) actually provides more color contrast and a more striking effect than highlighting. And, like highlighting, you will have the convenience of infrequent touch-ups that are necessary about every three to four months.

There have been many improvements in at-home streaking kits. It's easier now to pick the right kit for your shade of hair and never go wrong with the timing of the lightening process. There are kits for brunettes, blondes, and redheads—no longer is there only one kit for all shades.

The cap is the most common method of streaking hair. This clear, soft plastic headpiece is designed with little holes punched all over it (sometimes you have to punch all the holes). The trick here is to separate the strands to be lightened or colored by pulling them through the holes in the cap with a little gadget that resembles a crochet hook. It's easy but it does take a bit longer than many other haircolor procedures. I definitely recommend asking a friend to help you with all the hole punching and strand pulling. It will go more quickly, and those hard-to-get-at areas will get precision coverage.

There are also special effects kits available like Hair Painting, Light Effects, and Frost 'n Tip. All of these are forms of streaking. They are termed "special effects" because the color is placed on certain sections of the hair rather than throughout the entire head. Hair Painting uses a brush to lighten selected strands; Light Effects and Frost 'n Tip kits use a plastic cap during the application.

Reading the Box

Let's start with an important fact to remember. *Read the box before you proceed!* Actually, this is the most important thing you'll have to remember after selecting the right product.

You would be surprised at how many women don't read the instructions on the box or choose not to follow them. They prefer instead to use their own applications, timings, etc. That, of course, is when things go awry. Just do exactly what the manufacturer recommends.

You should also know that the shade pictured on the box front is not necessarily the shade you'll get on your particular hair. This picture shows the color as it has been done on pure white virgin hair. To learn what that color will look like on your natural color, read the chart on the back of the box. It will state exactly what you can expect from this particular shade on your hair. Easy!

Here's a tip that will really help you quickly understand more about the shade you are selecting. On the front of the box, you'll see the *number and name of the formula*. Just below that, you'll see the generic or general description of the shade that will help you visualize the shade shown on the box front. Turn the box over, look for the *Shade Selection Chart,* find your own natural color, and then see how this formula will affect your hair.

A medium ash blond shade, for example, may leave blond or white hair exactly as the box shows—a medium ash blond. But if your hair is light brown, this formula may leave your hair a lighter brown or a dark ash blond.

Finally, most at-home haircoloring products either contain everything you need to do color, or state what additional items you may need that are not included in the package. These items usually include a plastic applicator bottle, a separate bottle of developer, and other common items that are found in every store.

So, let's review:

1   You have read all the copy on the front and back of the box and seen that by following a few easy instructions you can color your hair at home.

2   You have studied the color of the hair on the box front,

looked at the number and the name of the formula, learned the generic description of the shade itself, and looked at the chart on the back to see what color *your* hair will turn out.

Once you open your package of haircolor, you'll note that the manufacturers suggest taking a patch test and a strand test to guarantee safety and satisfactory color results. I think these are important precautions—please take the few minutes required to do them.

The Patch Test

Certain people may be allergic to foods, drugs, cosmetics, or other items normally considered harmless. Allergies can sometimes develop suddenly. You could have been nonallergic to something last week and suddenly find yourself allergic to it now. That's why you *must* take this patch test for sensitivity twenty-four hours before each and every application. You can preview your new haircolor at the same time. Here are the instructions for a simple patch test.

1 *Prepare a test area.* With mild soap and water, wash an area about the size of a quarter behind either ear or on the inside of your elbow. Pat dry.

2 *Apply test mixture.* Shake the bottle four or five times. Measure one teaspoonful of the product you are using. With a cotton swab, apply a few drops of the mixture to the test

area. Use the remaining portion to do a strand test at the same time (see pages 80–82); this is how you test or preview color results on a strip of hair.

3   *Let dry.* Leave test area uncovered and undisturbed for twenty-four hours. If there are no adverse reactions, go ahead and color your hair.

If you do notice any reddening of the skin, burning, itching, irritation in or around the test area, you are allergic to the product and must not use it. It is at this point that I would consider talking to a professional haircolorist to see if there is another type or brand of haircolor to which you will not have an allergic reaction.

Consider also the fact that at certain times we may be allergic to a particular haircoloring; at other times, we may have no reaction to that same product. Certain medication we may be taking, for instance, can affect our reaction to haircoloring. There are also other factors that your haircolorist can explain to you.

Don't be discouraged by one allergic reaction. This does not mean that you can never color your hair again. Keep trying, and let the experts help you make that choice.

The Strand Test

The strand test, also known as the preview test, is a wonderful feature of modern haircolor and a very helpful step for a beginner with at-home color. This important test literally allows you to preview how the color will turn out on a little snip of hair you've clipped from the back section of your hair.

Here are the three basic steps of the strand test.

1 *Snip Several Hair Strands.* Snip several strands of hair close to your scalp (one-quarter inch wide) from the darkest part of your hair usually located way in the back of the head (at the nape). Tape the strands together at one end.

2 *Apply Color and Time.* Place the strand into the color mixture left over from the patch test. Make sure the hair is completely covered. Start timing.

3 *Wipe Clean and Check.* After twenty minutes, wipe the strand clean, let it dry, and check the color. If it's not the shade you want, return the strand to the test mixture and check every few minutes until it is the right shade. If, after forty-five minutes, the strand is not the shade you want, you may need a different haircolor shade. If you desire to cover gray and the color isn't doing the job sufficiently, try leaving the test strand in the color mixture for an additional ten minutes.

Remember that timing is extremely important to obtain satisfactory haircolor results. Though many products now have a built-in timer when color stops developing, it is still vital that you closely follow the timing of any step. In some cases, you may find that you like the color results when allowing less time than the directions say; your strand test will tell you this. Otherwise, follow the manufacturer's directions. But don't be afraid to experiment a bit . . . nothing drastic will happen. That's the fun of haircoloring today.

Setting Up for Haircolor

Lighting is the most important factor to consider when you're setting up for haircolor. I usually recommend either the kitchen or the bathroom depending on the strength of the lighting.

The ideal lighting situation is a combination of natural and overhead lighting. You will usually find this type of lighting in an area near a window. This reflects your color in its truest sense.

In my salon, the floor reflects lots of natural sunlight emanating from big picture windows. Other than that, I have special built-in overhead spots to illuminate the top of the hair when I look down to do color on my clients.

If you have flourescent lighting, remember that this alters or modifies the true colors of your hair. This type of lighting often imparts a greenish or blueish effect on both hair and skin. It has a drabbing effect which can slightly throw off your eye for color.

Find a comfortable spot to sit or stand near a big mirror. And ask a friend to help you work on areas of the head that are difficult for you to see and reach.

YOUR COMPLETE HAIRCOLORING CHECKLIST

As a professional hair colorist, I always try to work as neatly and be as organized as possible. By getting together all the things needed at once, and having all your materials within arms' reach, you will be ready to go ahead with comfort, confidence, and control. It's much like working in your kitchen, whipping up a casserole or baking a beautiful cake for a special occasion. You gather together all your ingredients, follow the recipe as best you can, and then enjoy the great results.

Remember that *timing is a key factor* in both cooking and coloring—pay very careful attention to the timing of your haircolor procedure. As you know, all the right ingredients in the world won't help if you burn the dinner—or, in this case, overprocess your haircolor beyond the manufacturer's recommended timing.

Now, review the few simple items you will need for easy at-home haircoloring and gather them all together. Have fun!

- ☐ Rubber/plastic gloves (usually contained in package).
- ☐ Timer.
- ☐ Plastic cape.
- ☐ Cold cream (or vaseline).
- ☐ Plastic applicator bottle (sometimes not in package).
- ☐ Small plastic mixing bowl (usually in kit).
- ☐ Highlighting brush (usually in kits but size of brush is limited; for a wider applicator brush, try an artist's supply store).
- ☐ Highlight/streaking cap (available in most kits).
- ☐ Towel for shampooing.

- ☐ Scissors (to snip a bit of hair at the back for strand test).
- ☐ Haircolor stain remover (specially developed liquid cleanser to remove unwanted haircolor stains around hairline . . . like Metalex or Sea Breeze).
- ☐ Haircolor developer (the liquid or creme agent that activates color process when combined with color in bottle; often sold separately).

Before You Begin . . . Some Final Thoughts

Remember, when you color your hair at home, you should always use a fresh mixture. Don't use leftovers. Haircoloring that has been opened and saved, for even a short time, loses its potency and won't give you the results you wanted.

After you have colored your hair, remember, too, that it's going to take a few days for your final color to blend and "settle," a process called oxidation. Only then will you be able to appreciate the true fullness of the color and how it "took" to your hair.

Also, give yourself some time to adjust to this newer you. If you get the urge to "just add a little more" or make other adjustments, wait a while after your last application. You may not want "a little more" once your color has had a chance to oxidize to its final richness and hue.

Chapter 5

"How-to" At-Home Techniques

Applying All Haircolor . . . Where to Begin and End

No matter what type of haircolor method you're using you should always begin and end in the same sections of the head. This will give you a sense of order and organization which is just as important to the at-home colorist as it is to a professional. These are the steps you should follow:

1 You will always comb your hair into four basic sections—the left back, the right back, the left side, and the right side. Separate these sections with clips; this will allow you to work within each section in a neat, orderly fashion.

Color Your Life . . . With Haircolor

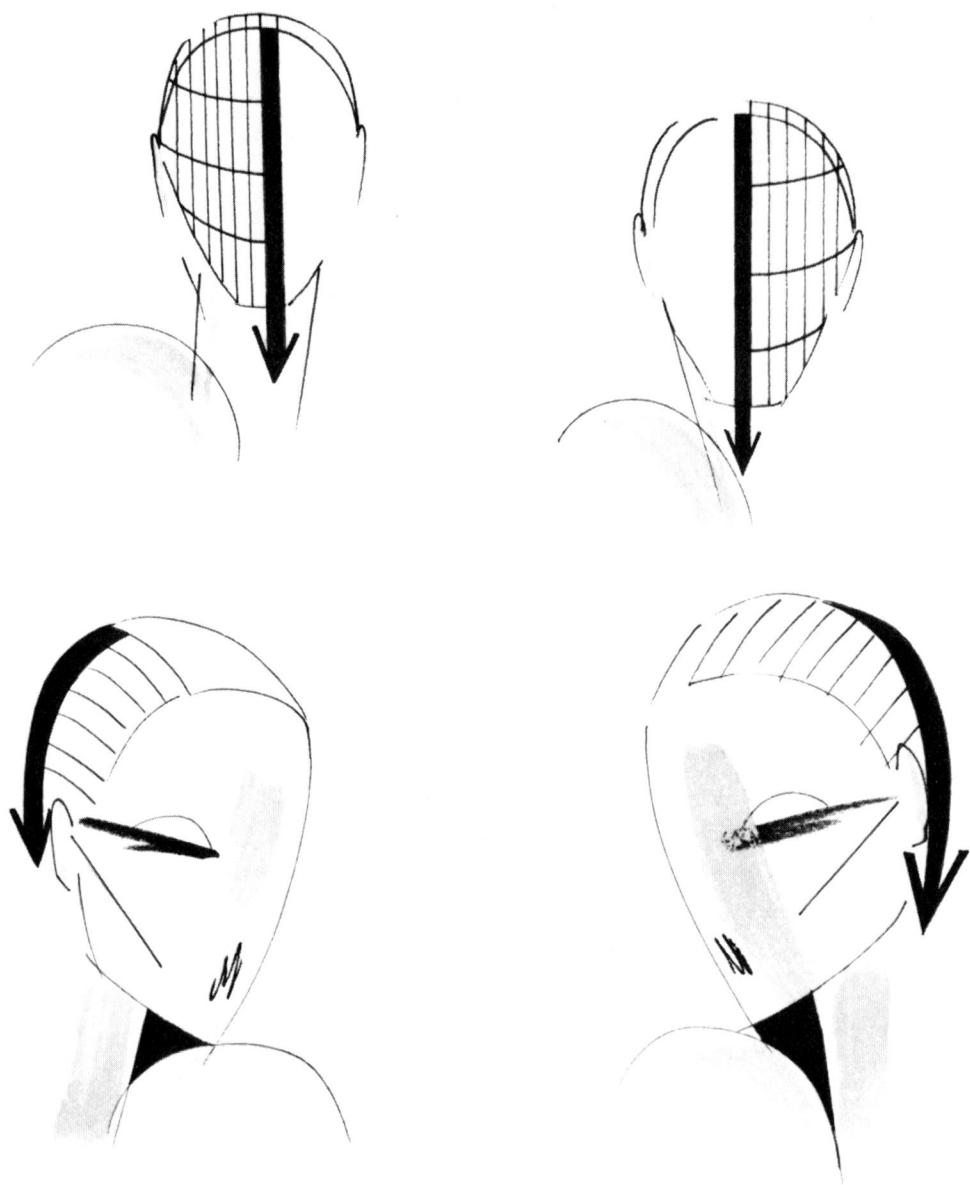

For all haircoloring, begin with the left back section and proceed to the right back, the left side, and finally to the right side.

2 Always start your color application in the back section, beginning with the left back and then the right back.

3 After completing the back sections, apply color to the left side and then to the right side.

It's so easy—this is all you have to remember when you do basic applications of semipermanent and permanent haircoloring. The following at-home techniques are creative alternatives to the standard "bottle application" technique.

Temporary Color Application

Temporary color is the easiest and fastest coloring technique. It's as simple as combing your hair. The color is applied to dry or wet hair, combed through, and left in. This is the most common way to apply temporary color. And there's no patch test involved.

If the color is in a styling gel base, the hair is styled first, and the color is "placed" in desired sections as you would apply an ordinary setting gel.

If you are using a color spray, simply style hair first and spray the color where you want to see it (see the tie-dyeing technique on pages 112–13).

Temporary colors can be removed easily by shampooing. They literally last until the next shampoo.

Semipermanent Color Application

Semipermanent color is my all-time favorite haircoloring technique because it adds shine and warmth to any head of hair, and has unique conditioning and coloring abilities. It is mistake-proof haircoloring.

Semipermanent color can be used on natural hair, hair with gray and hair that has been previously treated with highlights or one-process color.

Be sure that you have taken the patch test before applying color to damp, clean hair.

APPLICATION WITH BRUSH

1. Part hair into the four basic sections—left back, right back, left side, and right side. Use a clip to hold sections in place.

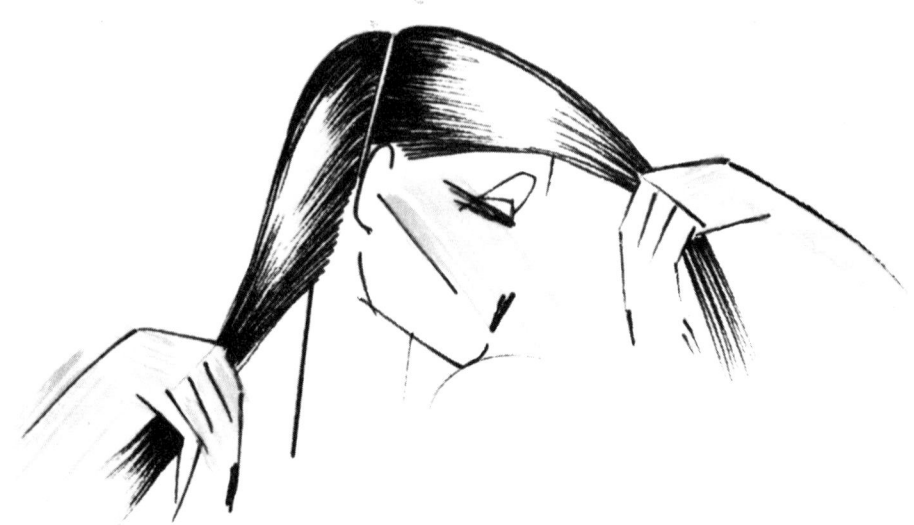

"How-to" At-Home Techniques

2 Put on plastic gloves.

3 To prevent any dripping or staining of skin from color mixture, apply cold cream around the hairline and adhere strip of cotton to the cream.

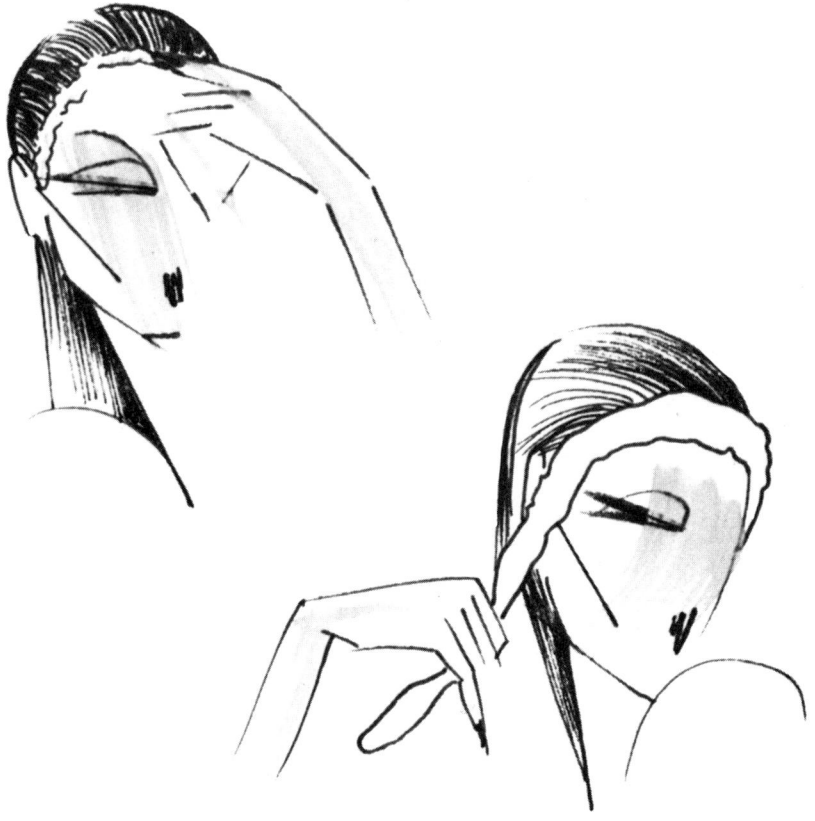

4 Mix formula according to manufacturer's directions.

5   To apply color, use the following method in all four sections of the head, starting with the back sections.

Using the tip of the applicator brush, take partings within each section as shown in the illustration; pull each small section straight out and away from the scalp, and brush on the color mixture from *root to end.*

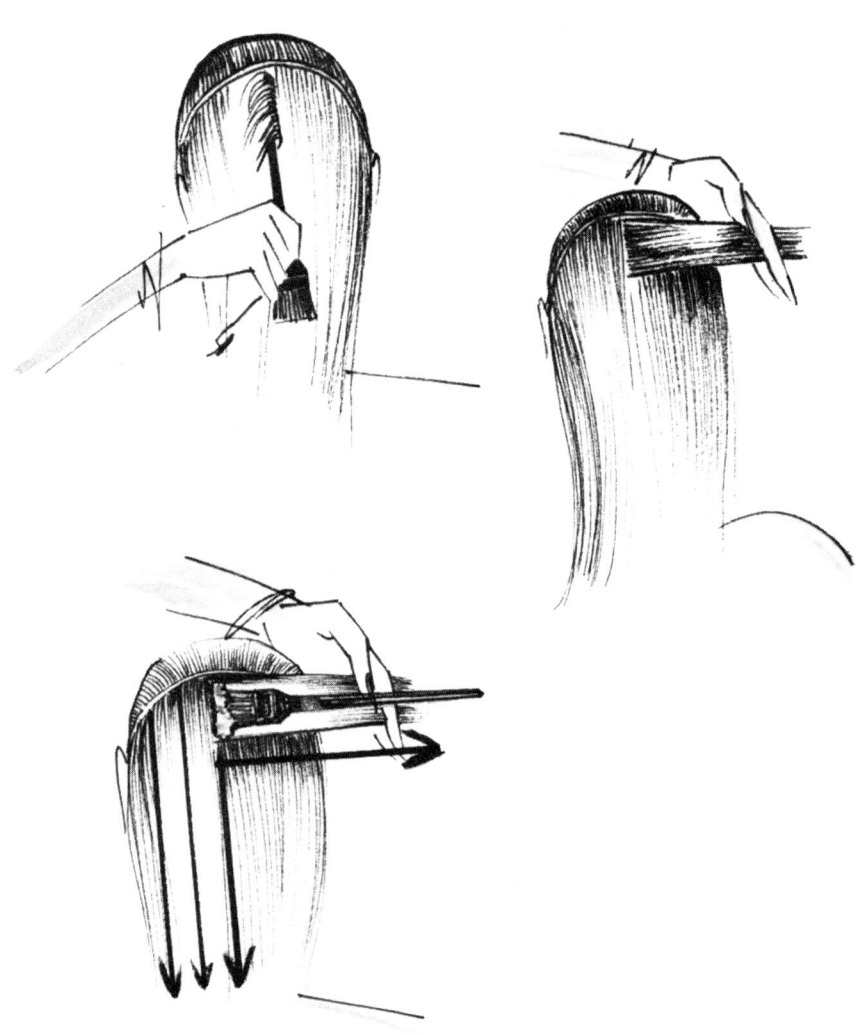

"How-to" At-Home Techniques

6   Now, with your fingers, gently work the color throughout the hair as if you were gently shampooing. Then smooth your hair back away from the face.

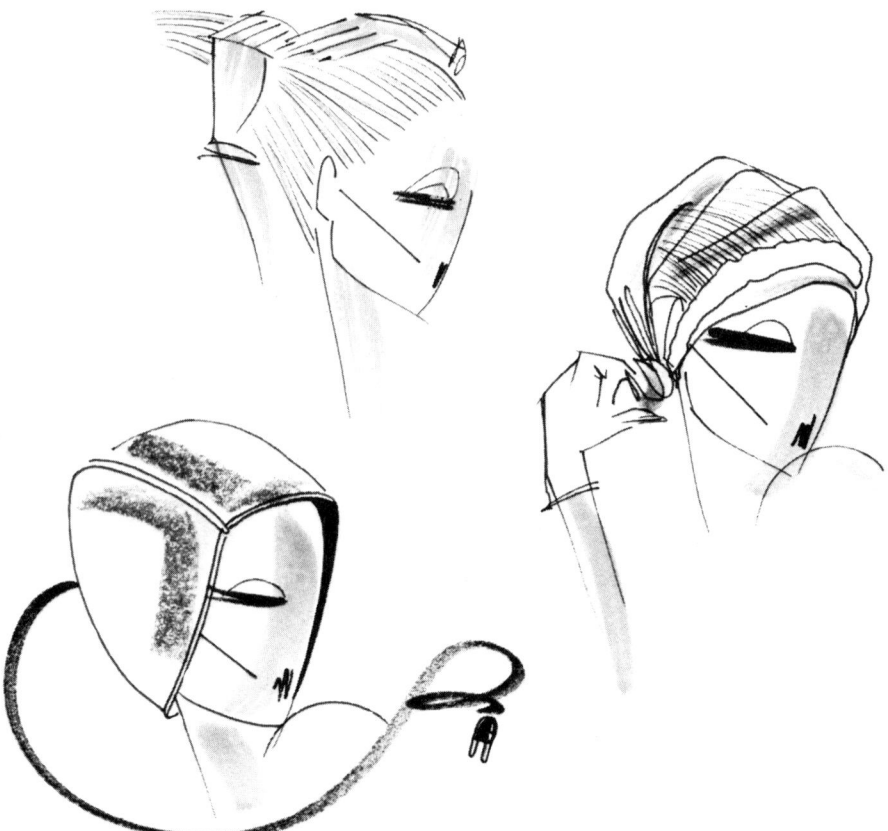

7   Cover hair with a plastic cap, and then a heating cap set on medium heat for about 30 minutes. *Set your timer.*

8   Rinse out thoroughly; condition and style as usual.

Permanent Color Application

This will give you the longest-lasting and richest depth of color. Permanent color is permanent—your hair will stay colored until it is cut off. And with this type of color, you can lighten, change your color family, and completely cover gray.

The permanent color method does require retouching the hair about every four to eight weeks depending on your rate of hair growth and how far you bring your new color from your natural shade.

The most common ways to apply permanent color are with a brush or with an applicator bottle. I prefer the brush technique because it offers more control and precision application for both the experienced and the beginning colorist.

The following steps will show you how to do a basic application on virgin hair (hair that has never been colored before), and then the necessary retouching of the regrowth area every several weeks. Hair should always be dry. Remember to take the patch test before every application.

"How-to" At-Home Techniques

APPLICATION WITH BRUSH ON VIRGIN HAIR

1. Part hair into the basic four sections—the left back, the right back, the left side and the right side. Use clips to separate sections.

2. Put on gloves.

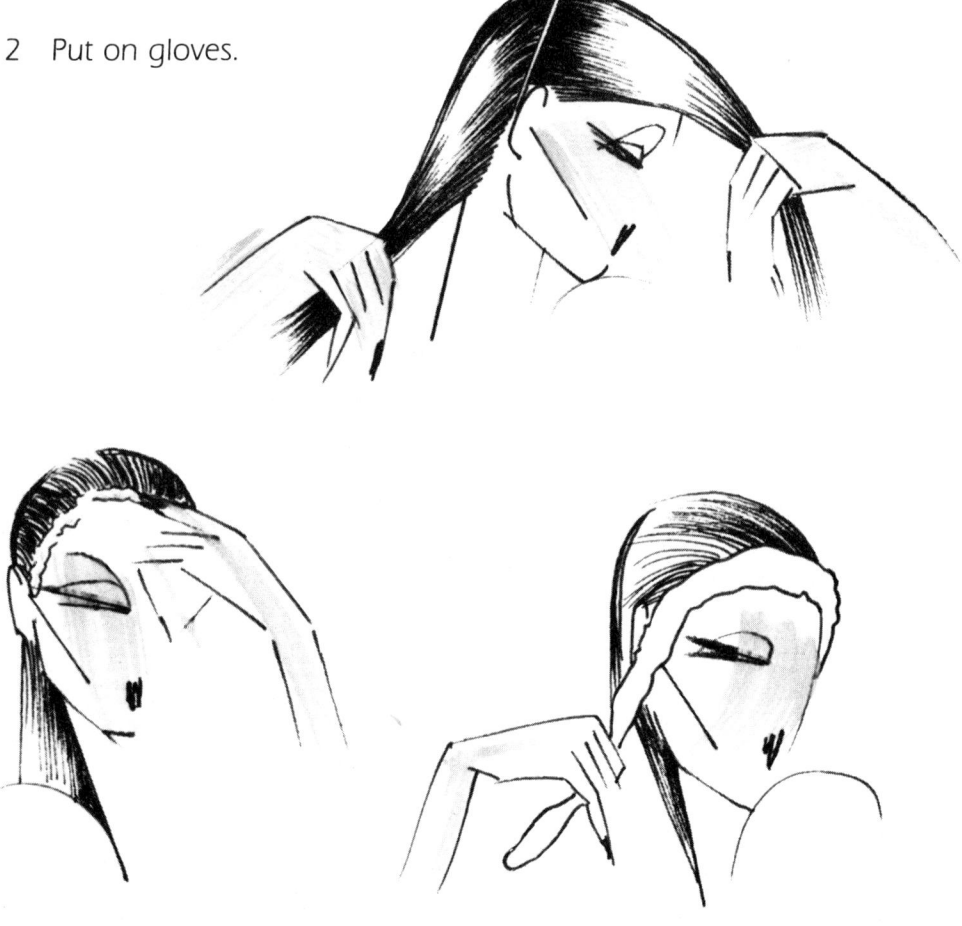

3. To avoid dripping or staining of skin by color mixture, apply cold cream around hairline and adhere cotton strip to it.

4   Mix formula according to manufacturer's directions.

5   To apply color, use this easy method in all four basic sections of the head, starting with the back: Using the tip of the applicator brush, take partings within each section as shown in the illustration. Pull each small section straight out and away from the scalp, and brush on the color mixture *starting about one-half inch from the root area out to the ends.*

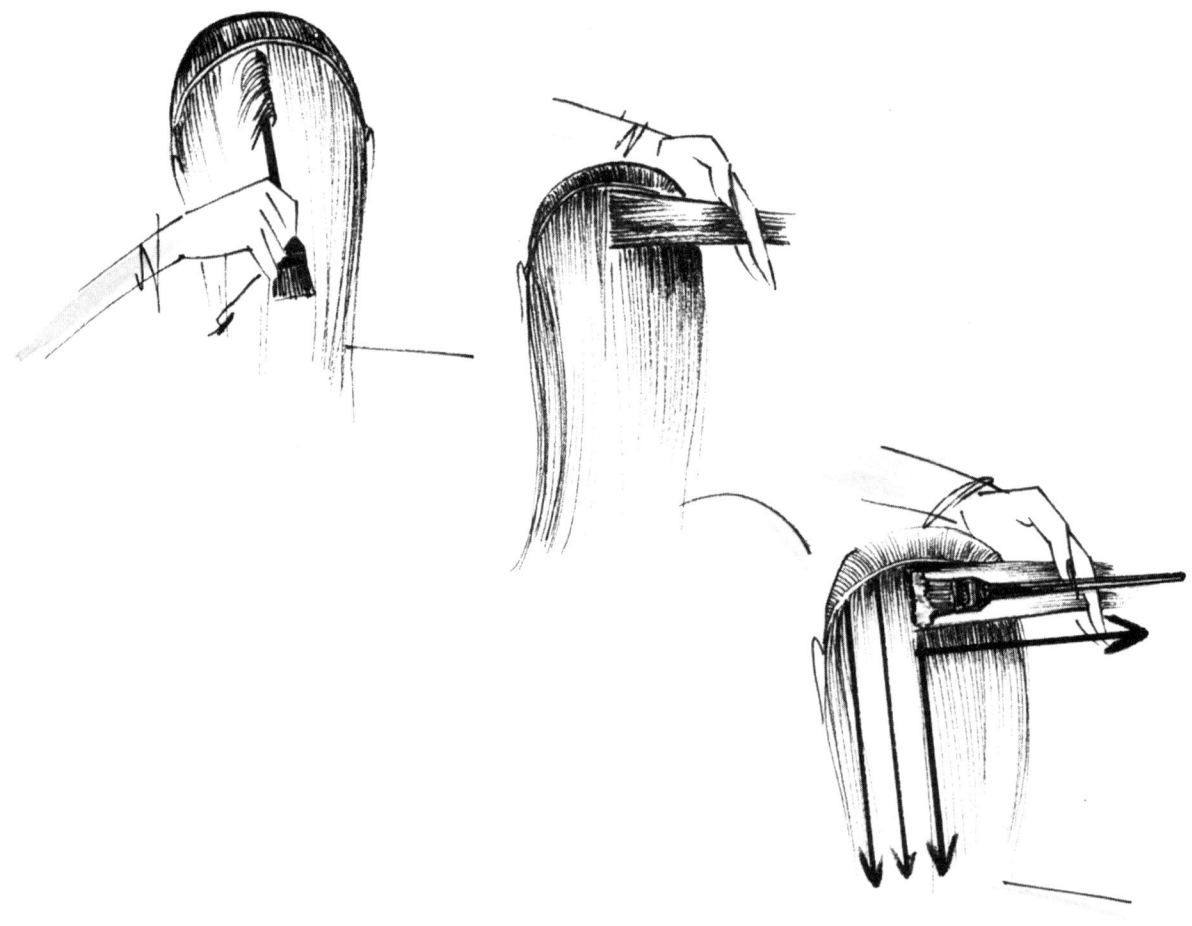

"How-to" At-Home Techniques

6 After completing all four sections of the head, let color develop about 15 minutes. *Set timer.*

7 When this 15 minutes is up, your objective will be to go back to all sections and apply the remaining color mixture only to the root area. Repeating the same order of sections and partings, use your brush to color the half-inch of hair at the roots. *Note:* You do the roots last because the color develops more quickly close to the scalp; body heat actually speeds up the color process.

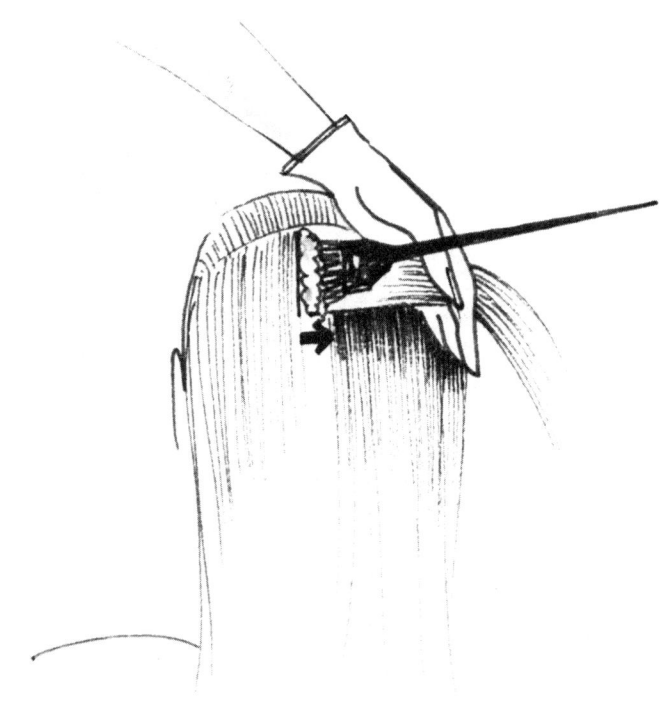

8 When all the roots have been covered with color mixture, let the roots and the rest of the hair develop for 15 more minutes. Your whole head now has color on it left to develop. *Set timer.*

9 When developing time is up, simply shampoo out mixture; condition and style hair as usual.

BASIC RETOUCH APPLICATION WITH BRUSH

Retouching haircolor means coloring the new growth that occurs about four to eight weeks after the initial application on virgin hair. This easy procedure enables you to blend the new growth area (roots showing your natural haircolor) with the ends and maintains the even look of color over the entire hair shaft.

Here is the most common retouching procedure to color the regrowth first and work the remaining color mixture through on the rest of the hair (this takes only about ten minutes to develop since it still retains the color from the basic application):

1 Part hair into the four basic sections—left back, right back, left side, and right side. Use a clip to hold sections in place.

2 Put on plastic gloves.

3 To avoid dripping or staining of skin by color mixture, apply cold cream around hairline and adhere cotton strip to it.

4 Mix color formula according to manufacturer's directions.

"How-to" At-Home Techniques

97

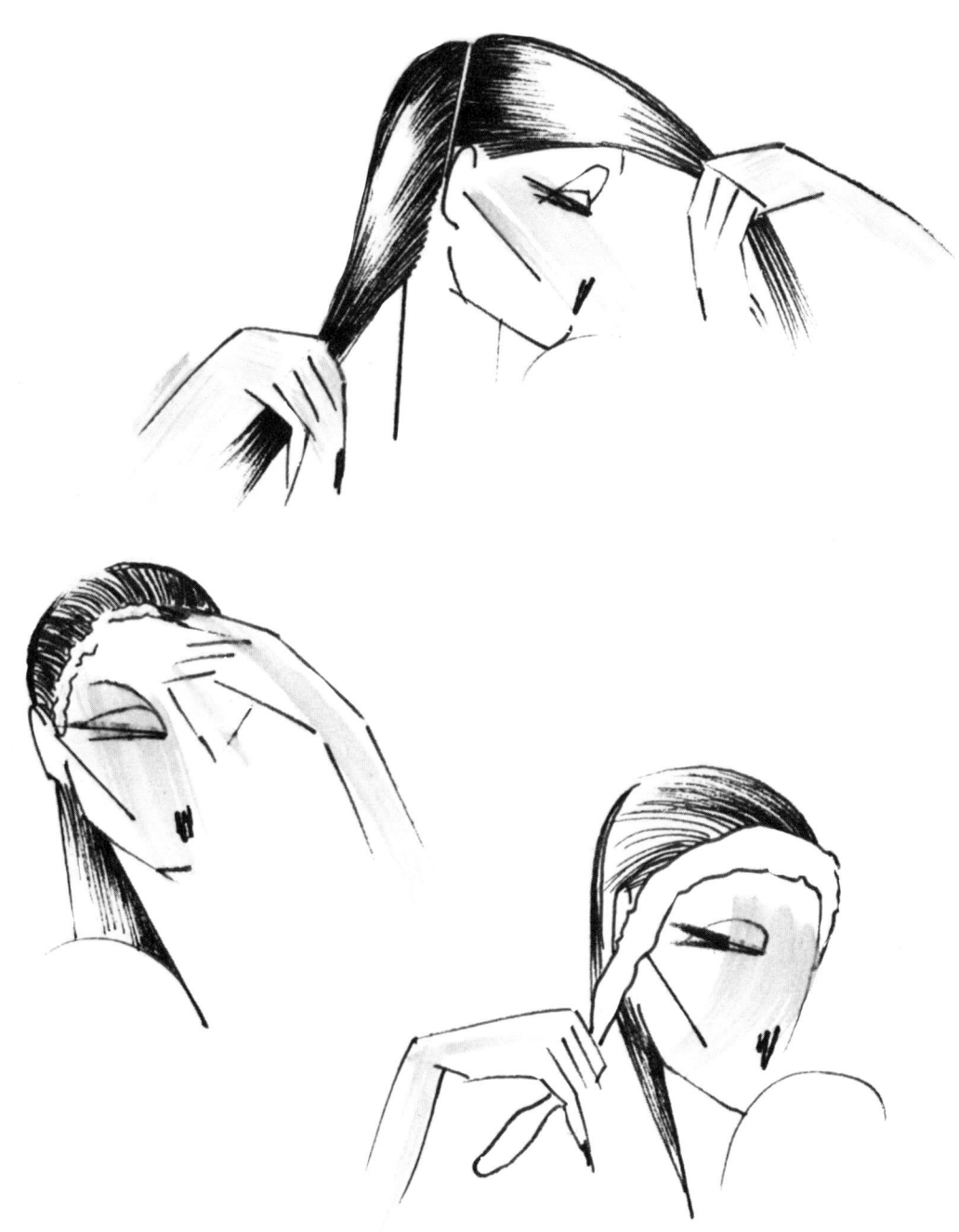

5 To apply color, use this method in all four basic sections of the head, starting with the back: Using the tip of the applicator brush, take partings within each section shown in the illustration. Pull each small section straight out and away from the scalp, and brush on the color mixture on the root area.

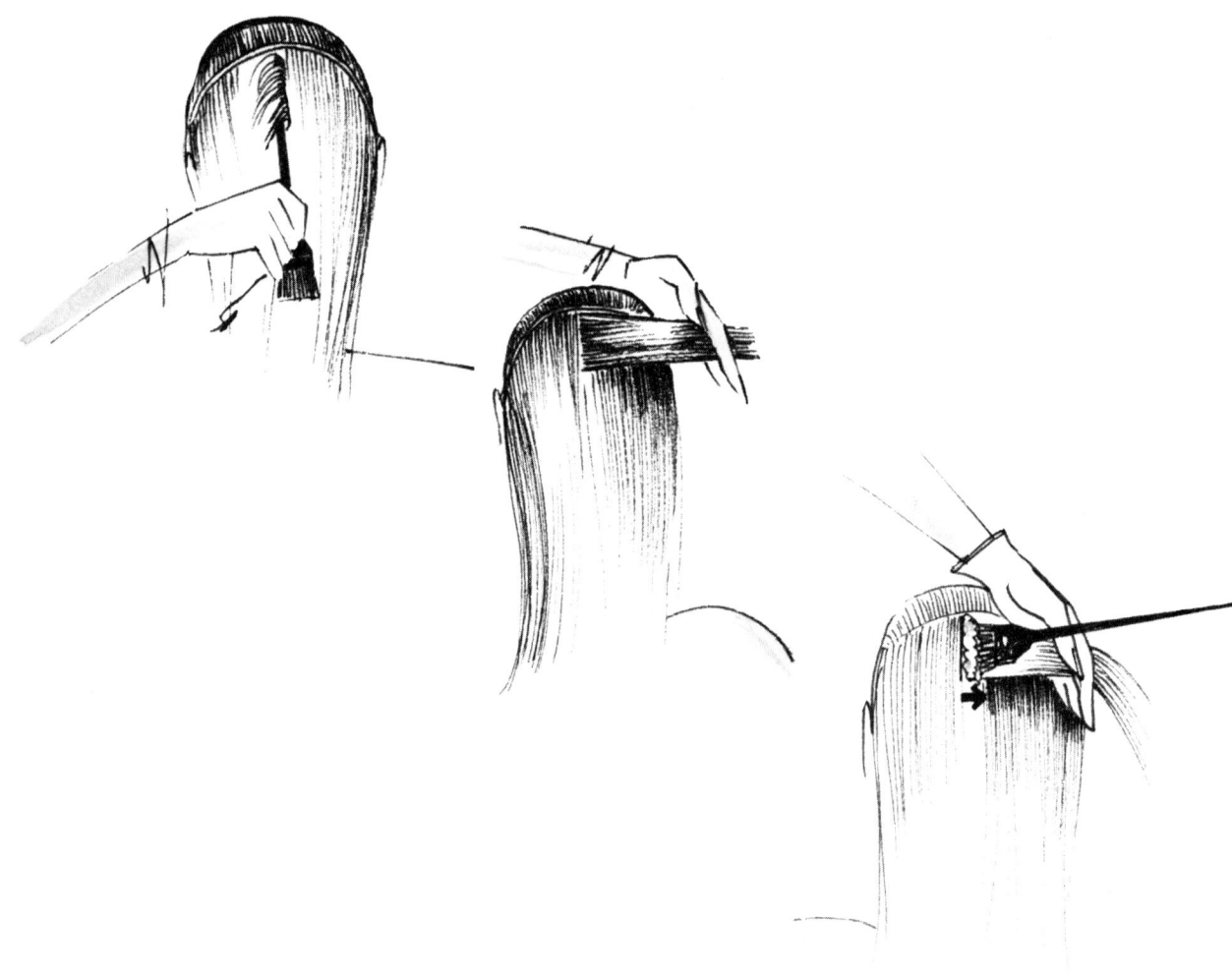

6   After completing all four major sections of the head, let the color develop at the roots for about 20 minutes. *Note: manufacturer's directions may suggest a different length of development time—use this as your guide. Set timer.*

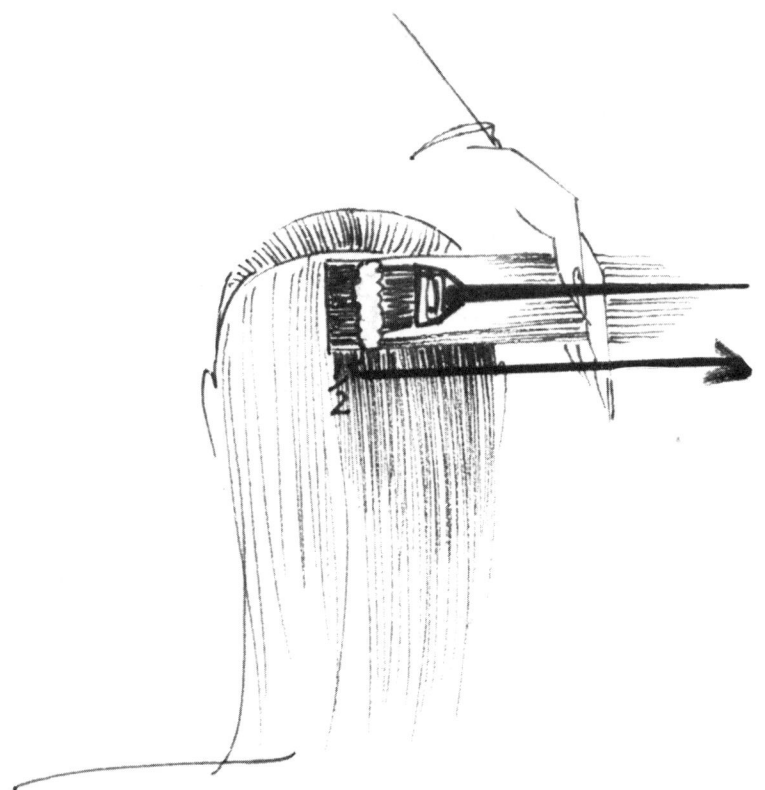

7   When this 20 minutes is up, your objective is to apply the remaining color mixture to the rest of the hair. Repeat the same order of sections and partings; use your brush to color the major part of the hair shaft that didn't get color applied earlier.

8   When hair in all the sections has been completely covered by the brush, gently work the color throughout the hair with your fingers as if you were gently shampooing your hair. Arrange the hair loosely and allow the color to now develop on *the whole head for another 10 minutes. Set timer.*

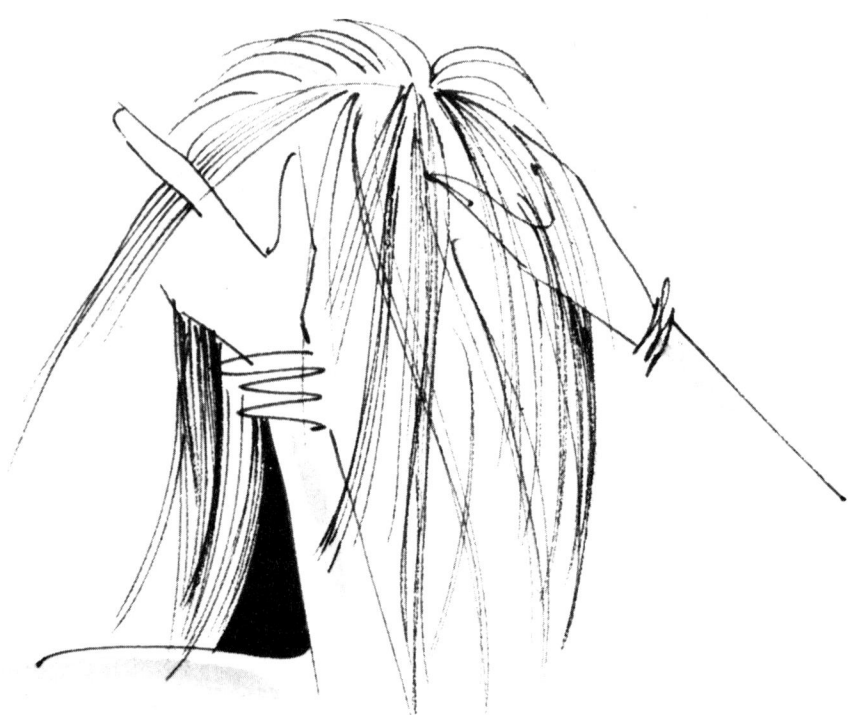

9   When development time is up, shampoo out color mixture; condition and style hair as usual.

BASIC RETOUCH APPLICATION WITH BOTTLE

I would recommend this technique for the experienced colorist. Basically, the procedure involves using the same bottle in which you mix your color formula to help you apply the color as well. I call this the old-fashioned "squeeze and smudge" technique of doing touch-ups at the root area. You squeeze the color out of the applicator bottle and smudge the color in with your fingers. Your hair should be dry when you begin retouching.

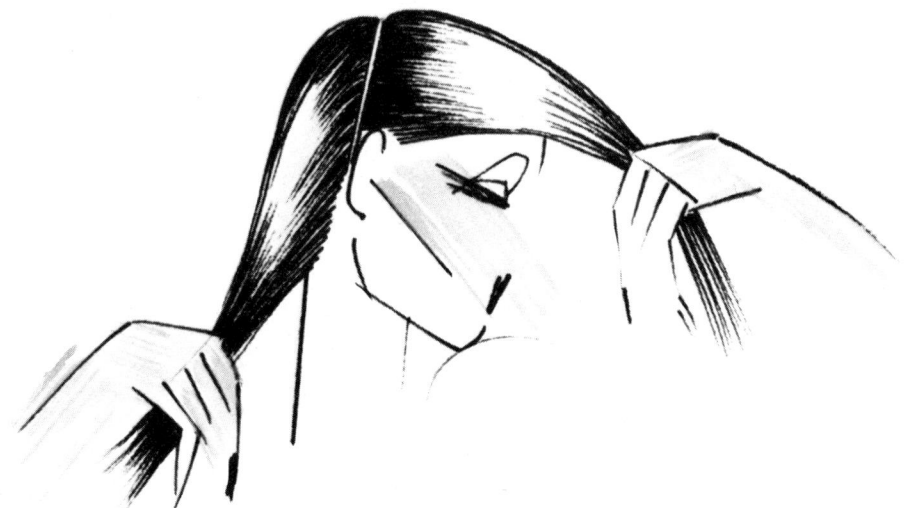

1. Part hair into the four basic sections—the left back, the right back, the left side, and the right side. Use clips to separate these sections.

2. Put on plastic gloves.

3   To avoid dripping or staining of the skin by the color mixture, apply cold cream around the hairline and adhere cotton strip to it.

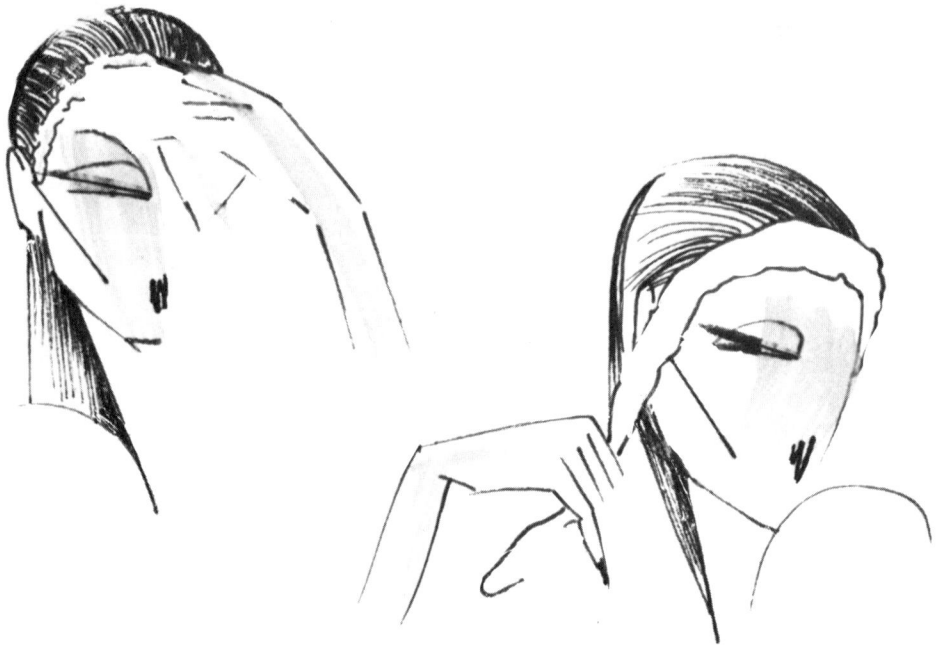

4   Mix formula according to manufacturer's directions.

5   To apply color, use this method in all four basic sections of the head, starting with the back. Use the tip of the *plastic applicator bottle* within each section shown in the illustration. Pull each small section straight out and away from hair; then squeeze out the color from the bottle to the root area. Use your thumb to "smudge" in the color at the roots.

"How-to" At-Home Techniques

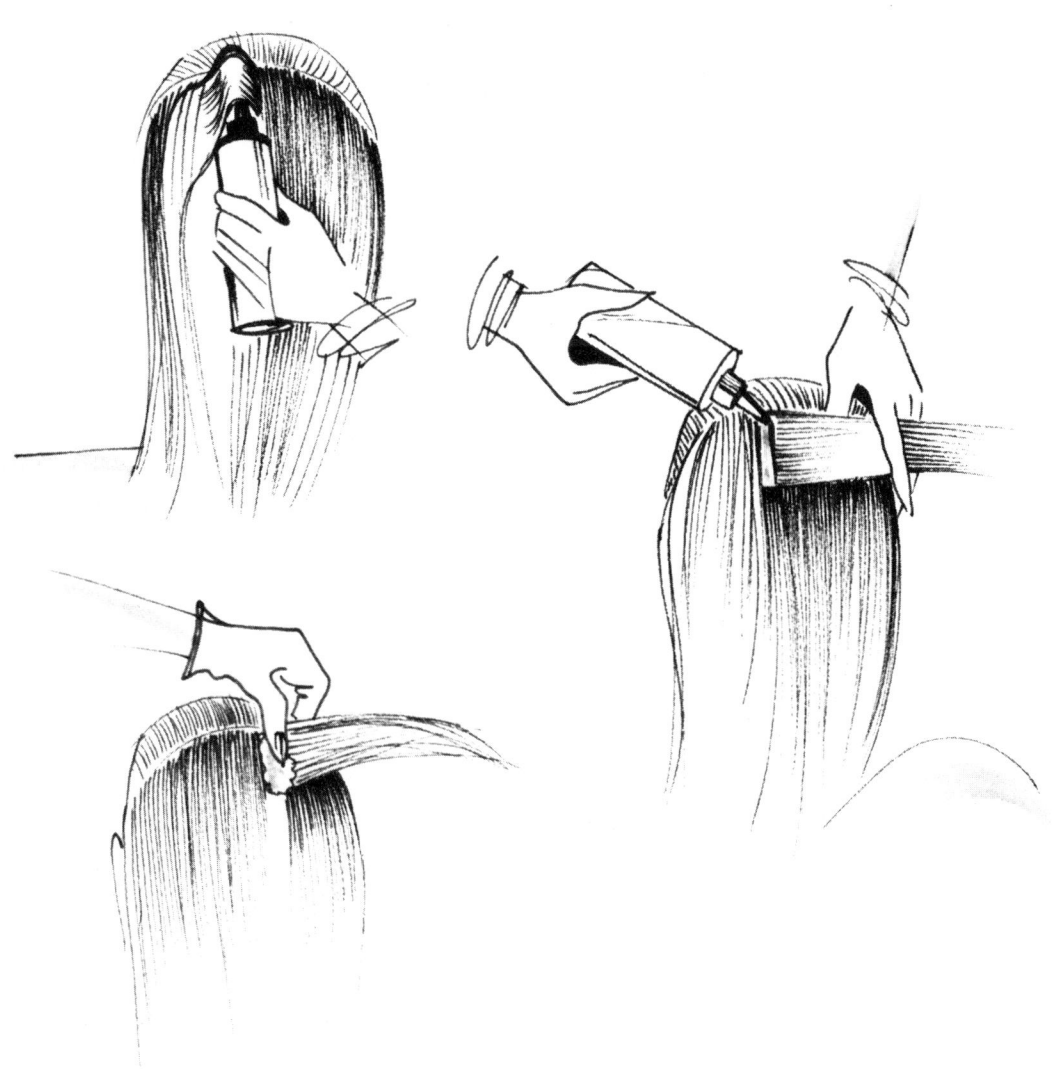

6 After completing all four major sections of the head, let the color develop at the roots for about 20 minutes. *Set timer.*

7 When this 20 minutes is up, your objective is to apply the remaining color mixture to the rest of the hair. Repeat the same order of sections and partings, squeezing color from the bottle along your small partings or sections; now use your thumb to smudge the color around the hair.

8 When hair in all the major sections has been completely covered by the tip of the applicator bottle and your fingers, gently work the color throughout the hair as if you were gently shampooing it. Arrange the hair loosely and allow the color to develop *on the whole head for another 10 minutes. Set timer.*

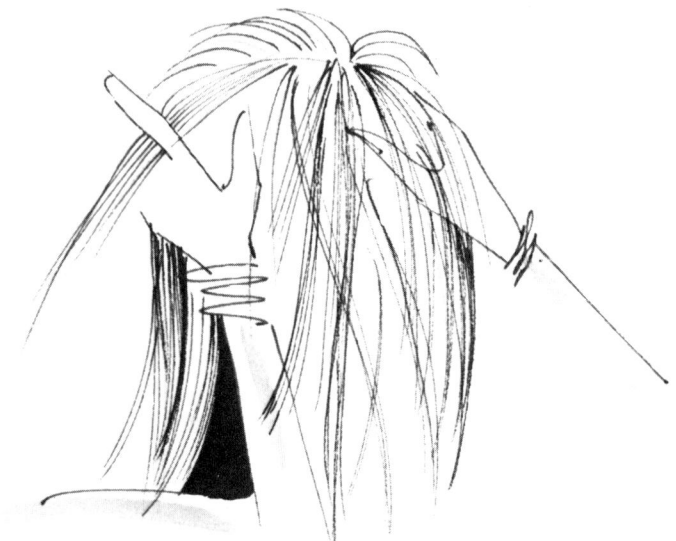

9 When development time is up, shampoo out color mixture; condition and style hair as usual.

Fine Basic Highlighting Using a Cap

For beautiful highlights exactly where you want them, the cap method of application will give you excellent control of placement. In fact, this is one of the most popular highlighting techniques in modern haircolor. I do recommend, however, that you ask a friend to help you the first time around because the technique involves pulling strands of hair through tiny holes in the cap. Hair should be dry during application.

There is quite a variety of highlighting kits on the market that use the cap method of application. I recommend Clairol's Frost 'n Tip kit.

1 Comb hair the way you usually wear it.

2 Put on plastic highlighting cap.

3 With "crochet hook" styling aid enclosed in the kit, pull about three or four strands of hair through each cap hole in the areas you want to lighten.

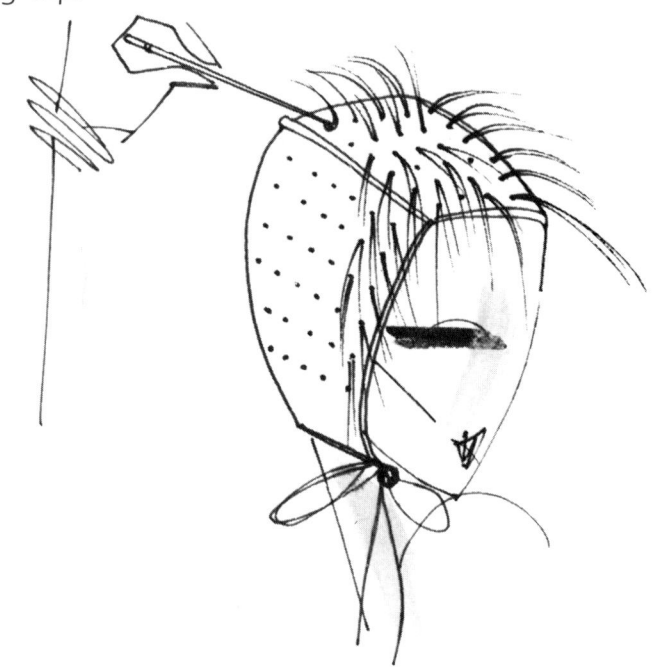

Color Your Life . . . With Haircolor

4   Put on plastic gloves.

5   Mix lightening mixture in enclosed plastic bowl.

6   Brush mixture all over exposed hair. Leave mixture on hair for the length of time specified in the manufacturer's instructions.

7   With a damp cloth, rub off some color from a few strands of hair to check the lightening process.

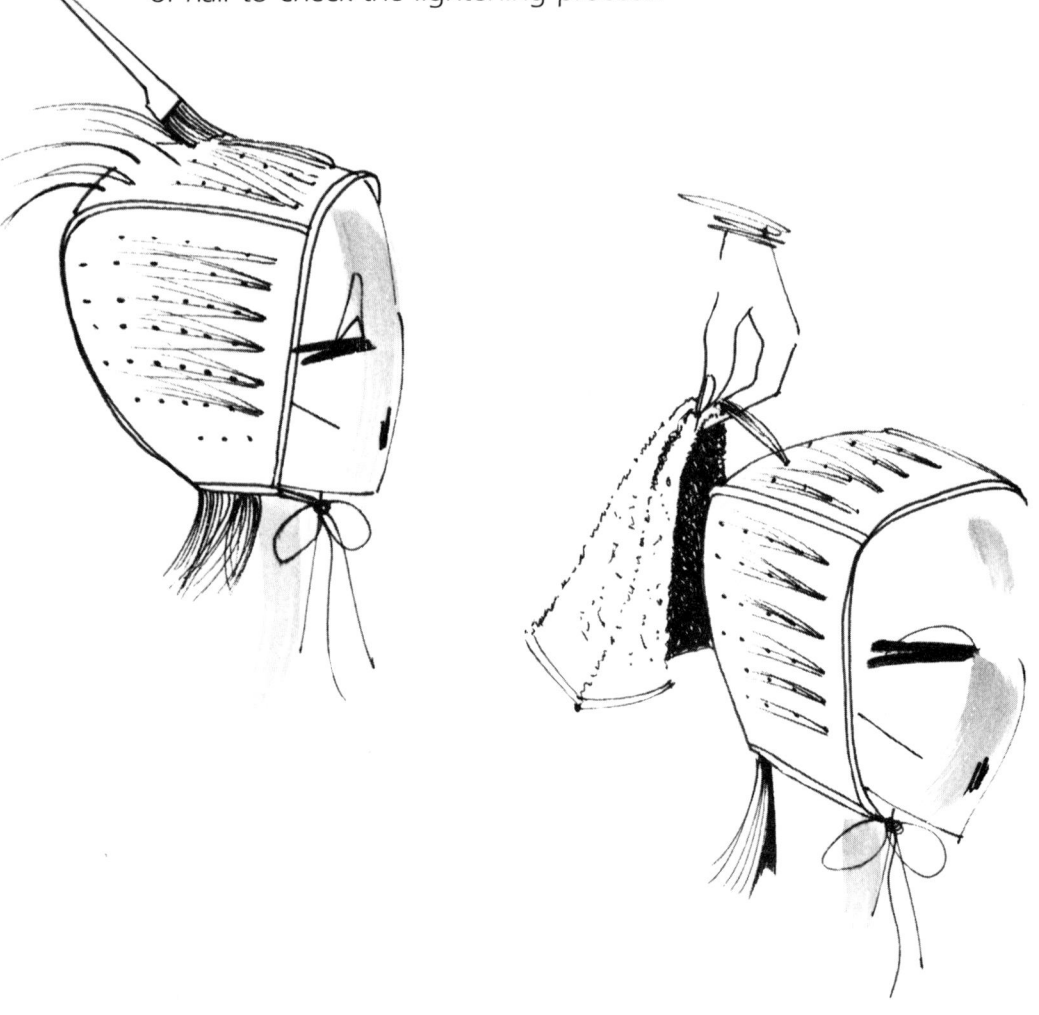

"How-to" At-Home Techniques

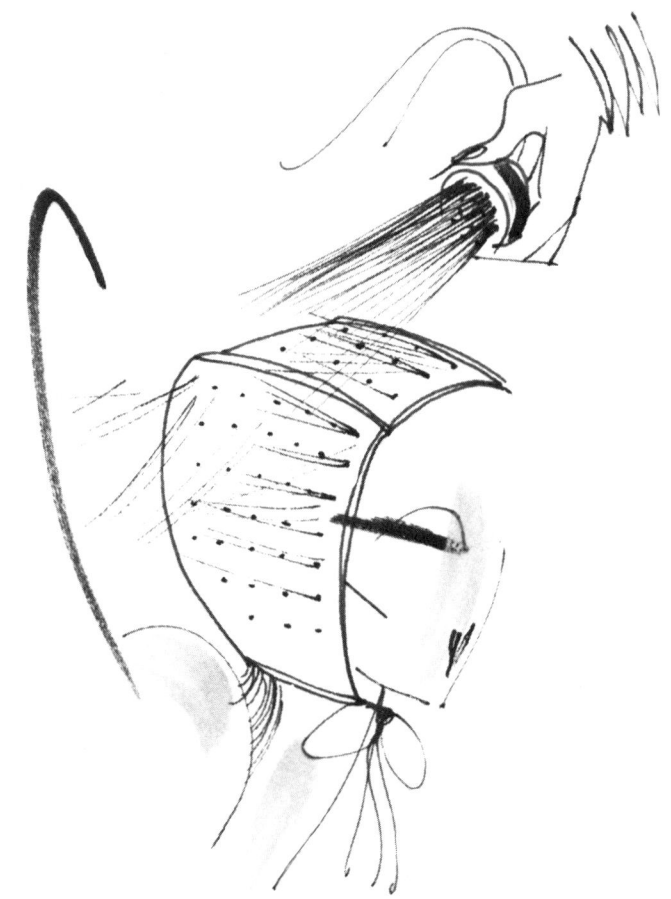

8   If the hair has reached the desired shade, rinse off mixture from all strands *while the cap is still on.*

9   Gently remove the cap.

10 Hair is now ready for shampooing, conditioning, and styling.

BASIC LOWLIGHTING WITH A CAP

An alternative to highlighting is lowlighting. Instead of lightening strands, you add depth for a more tone-on-tone effect.

Application
Follow the steps of basic fine highlighting exactly.

Recommended Color Mixture
Permanent color will give you lasting depth of color on the strands where you want it. I recommend that you mix it in a plastic dish with a thicker developer than you might normally use with a permanent color. For lowlighting, choose Clairol's White Creme Developer or Geloxide found in most stores.

Be sure to mix an amount of developer that equals the amount of color you're using. This will give you a good thick blend of color that is easy to apply with a brush—no color will seep down through the holes in the cap.

Hair Painting

This technique literally uses the art of painting—in this case, a lightening mixture on any area of the hair you wish. My favorite is Clairol's Hair Painting Kit.

There are several fashion looks that involve the hair painting technique. For instance, you can paint on soft edges of light along the bottom of bangs or along the bottom edge of longer hair—or outline the beautiful curls or waves of your hairstyle. I call this "tipping."

Another fashion look that involves painting your hair is silhouetting. As you would paint on a canvas, you creatively use your hair-painting brush to draw fine lines along only the surface of the hair—like the top and the crown areas where the sun would naturally lighten the surface.

Hair painting is always done on dry hair.

1 Comb hair into the style you always wear. *Note:* If you want to lighten only the tips or edges of your hairstyle, I suggest lightly teasing your hair with a comb; this causes the ends to stick up and be more visible.

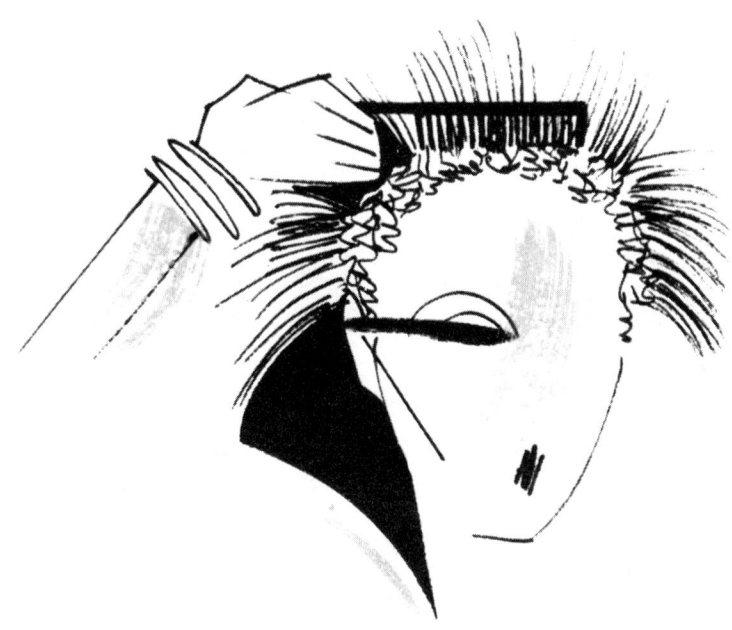

2 Put on your gloves.

3   Mix your creamy lightening formula according to manufacturer's instructions. This usually involves mixing the developer with a little packet of lightening powder included in the kit.

4   Brush or "paint" on the lightening mixture wherever you want it. This will be determined by which fashion look you choose to really accent your cut. Allow mixture to develop as indicated in directions. *Set timer.*

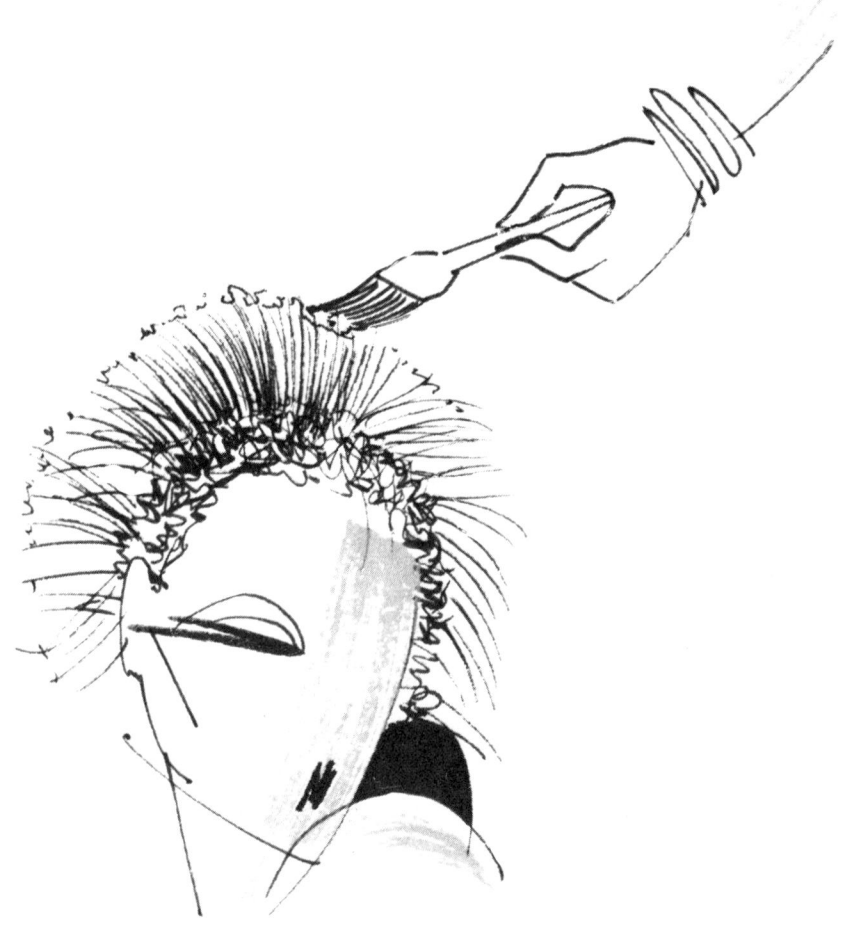

One fashion look of hair-painting is called tipping. This involves applying the lightening mixture to the tips or bottom of the hair, or along the curls.

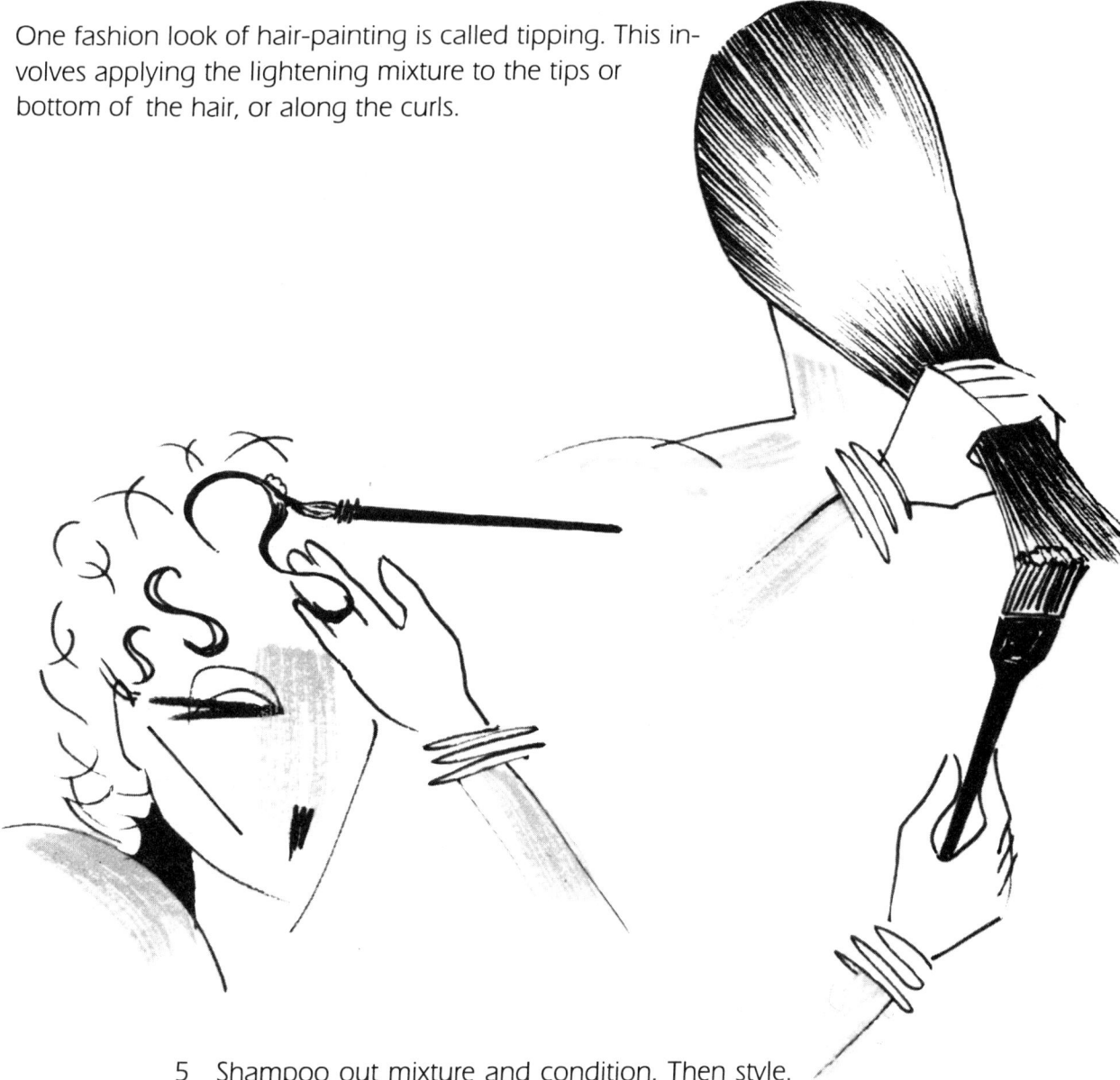

5   Shampoo out mixture and condition. Then style.

Tie-Dyeing

This is a favorite fashion look for longer hair. It creates soft "waves" or unique patterns of color that can be as bright or as subtle as you want. You will be spraying temporary color on your hair from a "mister" bottle, so choose temporary rinse in liquid form. Hair should be dry.

1   Arrange hair away from your face with your fingers so it falls softly down the back.

2   Beginning at the crown of the head, take a big section of the hair and fold softly; secure the section with a ribbon. Work your way from the crown section all the way down the length of your hair at the back, repeating the procedure.

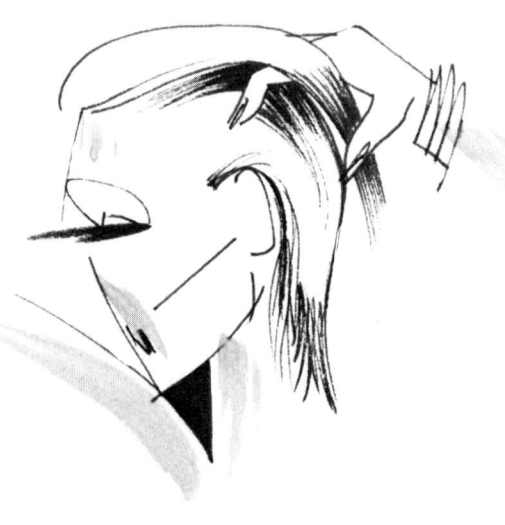
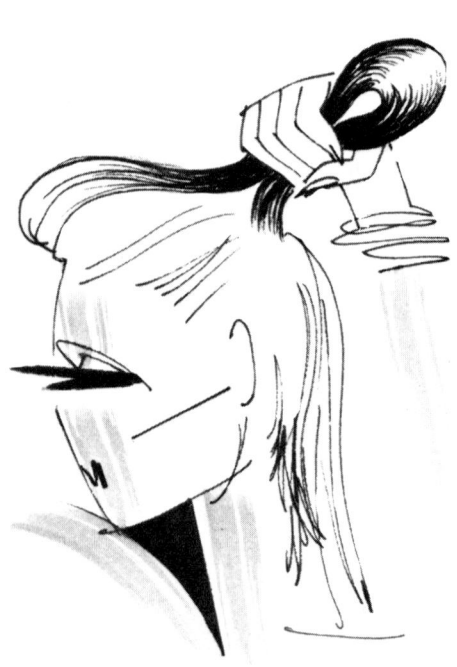

"How-to" At-Home Techniques

3   Put on plastic gloves.

4   Put your favorite temporary color rinse (liquid form) in a spray bottle and simply spray the ribboned sections only. *Note:* Be careful not to get color in your eyes or on your clothes.

5   Let the color dry—about 10 to 15 minutes.

6   Now, untie the ribbons and let this new color pattern in your hair turn a few heads at a party.

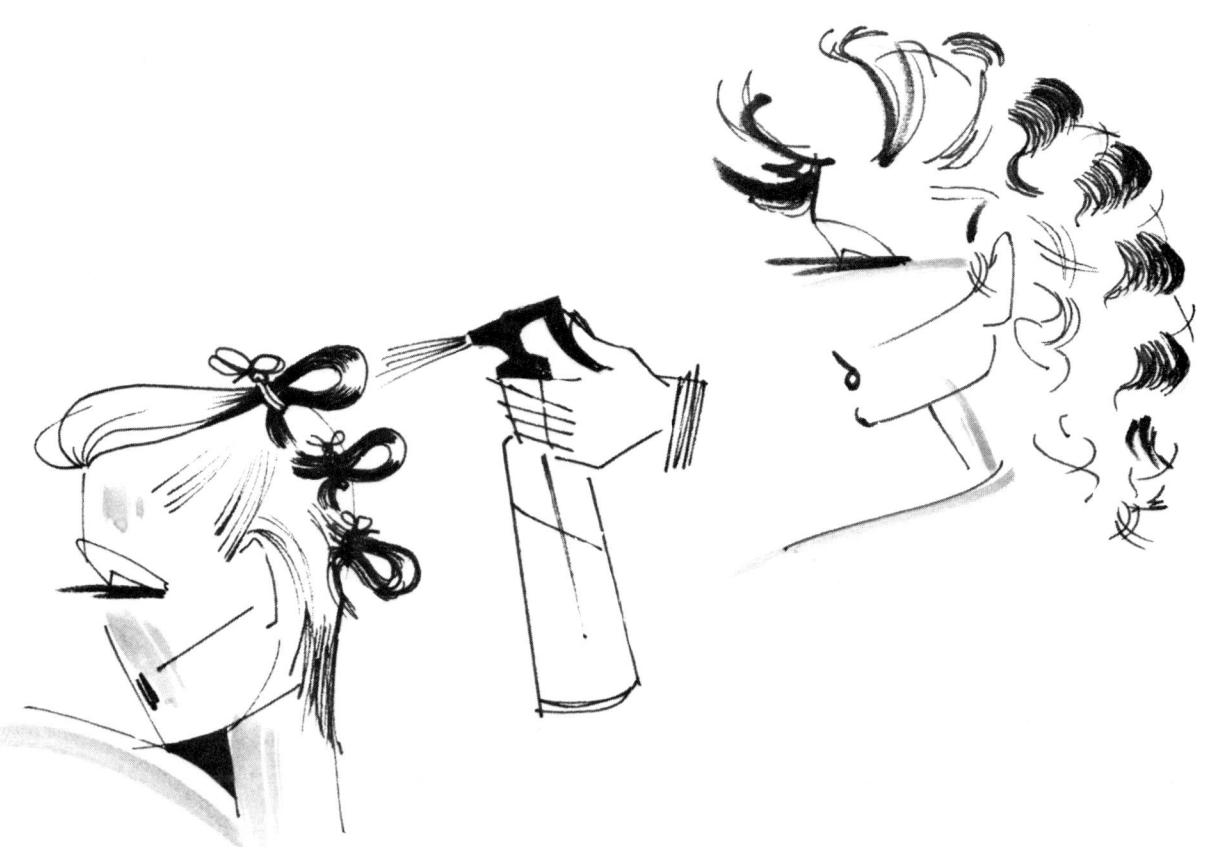

Color Blocking

Think of color blocking as sectional coloring—either lightening or adding color to whole sections or "blocks" of hair, like the back or the sides, to accent a particular cut. The effect is one of contrasting color on one head of hair, but instead of coloring just strands or doing allover color, we focus on one or more specific section(s) for a very dynamic effect. I always recommend using permanent color here for a lasting effect that won't fade away too quickly. Color can be applied on dry hair with either a bottle or a brush.

1 Comb your hair into the style you usually wear. Your objective here is to decide what section you want to lighten or color, and then clip back the rest of the hair so it won't get in your way. *Note:* I usually part the hair on an angle while separating or blocking sections to produce a very complimentary asymmetric effect.

2 Put on plastic gloves. Apply cold cream around the hairline of sections to be colored and adhere cotton strips to it.

"How-to" At-Home Techniques

3. Mix your color formula or lightening mixture according to manufacturer's directions.

4. Now, all you have to do is apply the mixture on the section you want with a bottle applicator or brush. Be sure to cover the entire area and all hair strands from root to end.

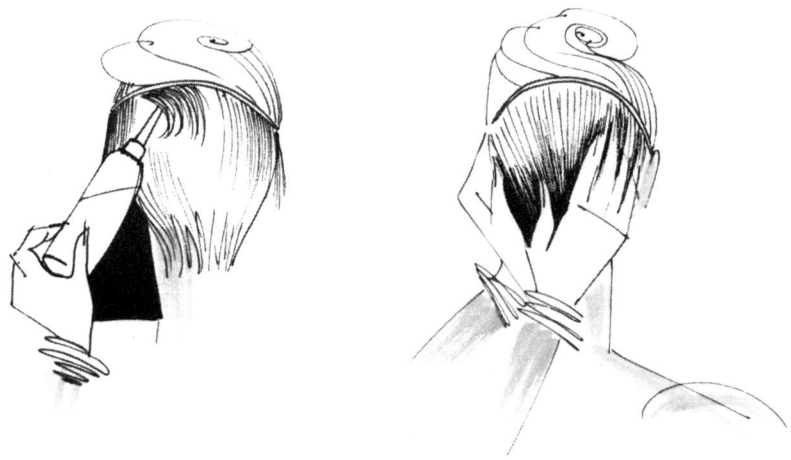

5. Work the color through the section with your fingers.

6. Let your color develop according to directions. *Set timer.* After 5 minutes, you may wish to preview the degree of color by toweling off some of the mixture from a few strands.

7. Shampoo out mixture; condition and style as usual.

How to Lighten Eyebrows

Sometimes our eyebrows look too heavy or dark. I often suggest lightening brows a shade or two to lighten up and "open up" the whole eye area. I recommend applying a permanent color with a brush or a Q-Tip on the brows only.

1. Begin by putting on your plastic gloves.

2. Mix your color formula with a thick creme developer (not a liquid) to keep the color mixture restricted to the brow area.

3. Carefully apply the mixture with a brush or Q-Tip and close the eye under the brow with which you're working. Let the color develop for about 3 minutes—no longer. *Set timer.*

4. Remove the color with a soft damp cloth. Be careful not to rub face or skin to avoid staining.

<u>CAUTION: DON'T GET COLOR MIXTURE IN YOUR EYES.</u>

So there you have it—easy at-home techniques anyone can master. By following a few basic steps it's now simple and fun to create the newest haircolor fashion effects.

"How-to" At-Home Techniques

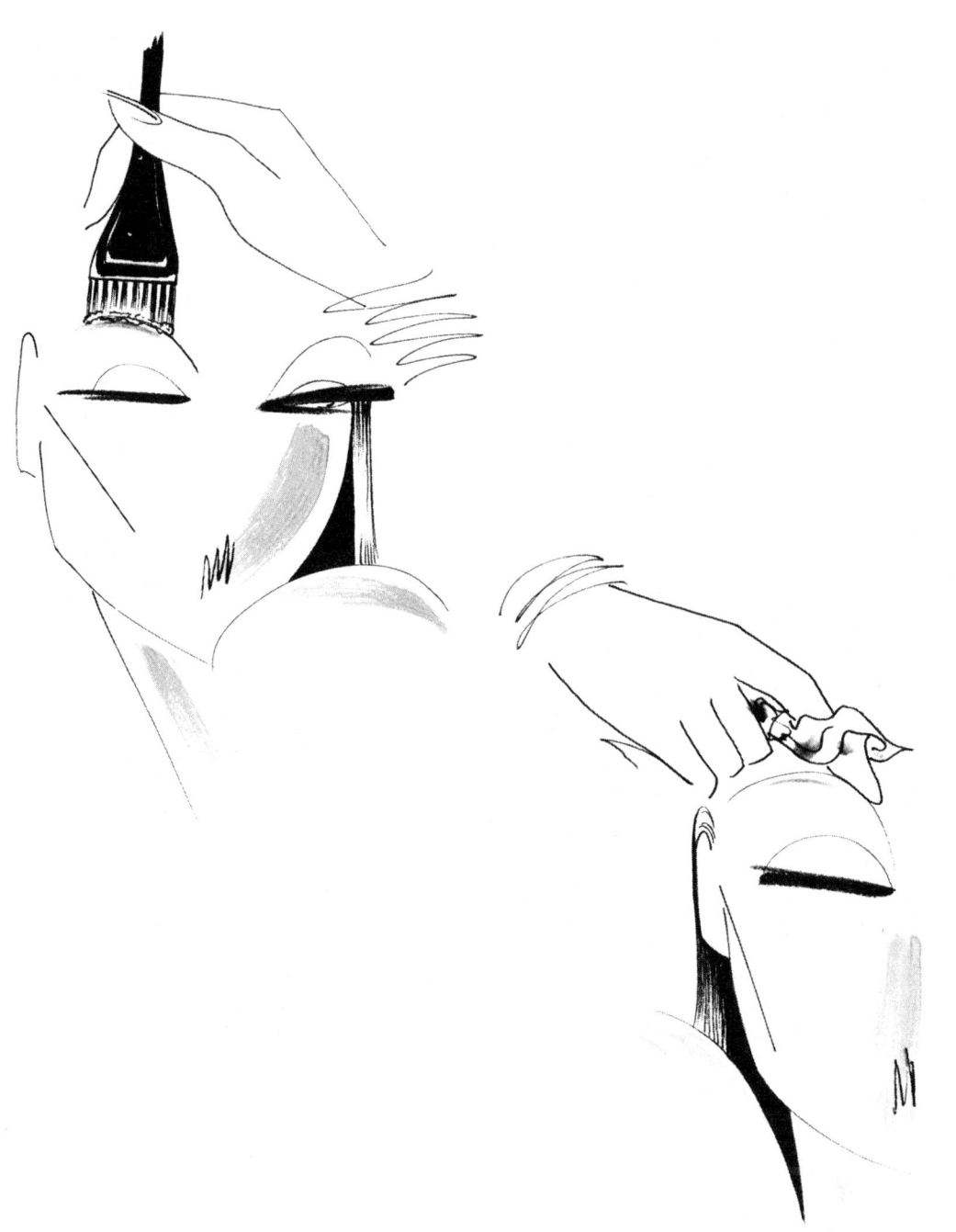

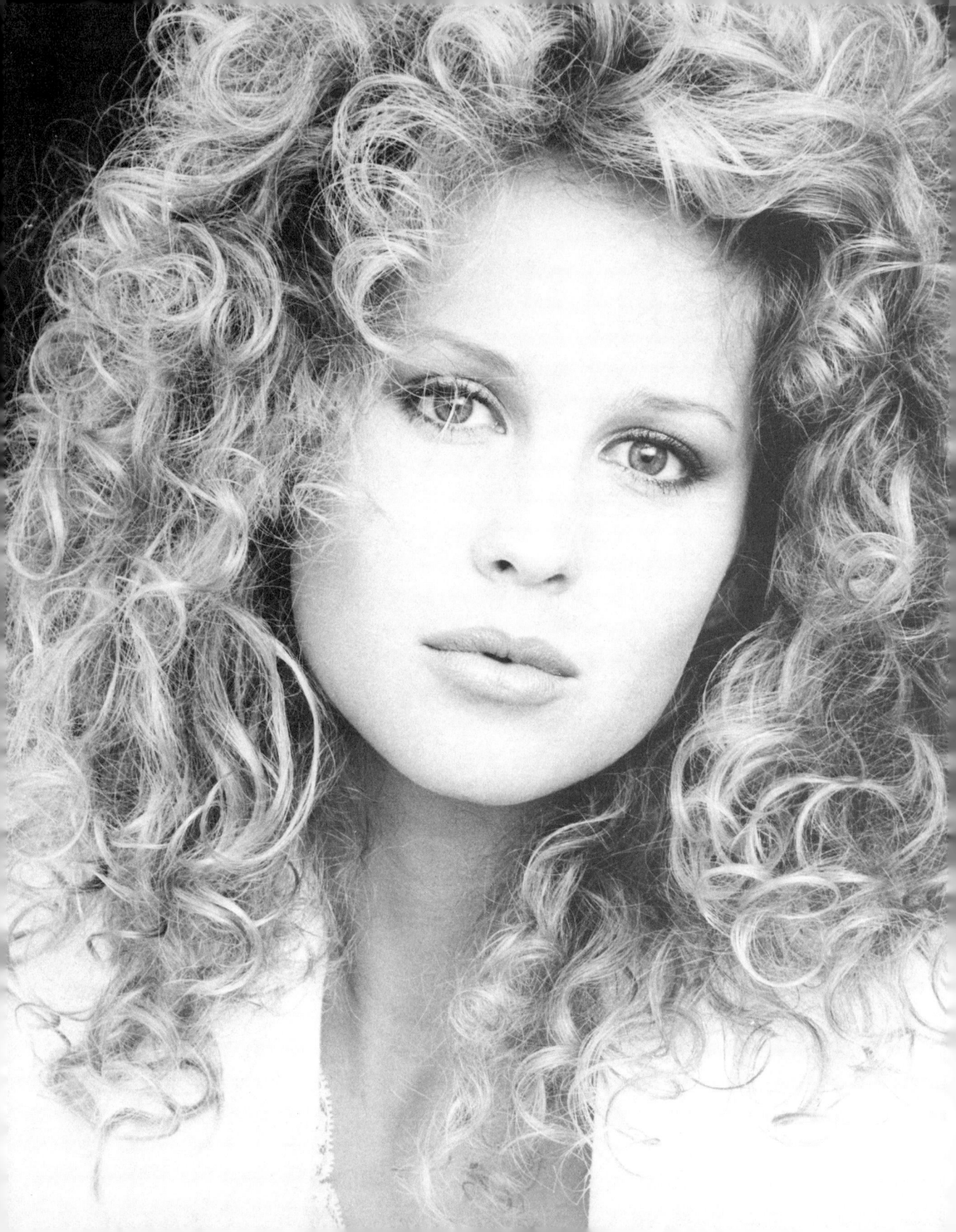

Chapter 6

Caring for Color-Treated Hair

Valuable Haircare Tips

Now that your hair is colored beautifully, there are just a few things to keep in mind to maintain that color, shine, and body.

1 Always keep your color looking fresh. Semipermanent color usually must be renewed after four to six shampoos. Allover color should be touched up about every four weeks. Highlighting needs refreshing only three to four times a year.

2 Keep color-treated hair shiny and clean, Dirt, oil, setting aids, and sprays coat the hair shaft and make the color look slightly duller or "off."

3 "Gentle handling" of your hair is another protective strategy. When you color your hair, you alter its texture. Your

hair actually has a fuller quality because coloring opens the cuticle on the individual hair shaft. This "open" texture makes hair more likely to "grab" on to other pieces of hair and thus tangle when washed. During shampooing and combing out, it is possible to cause some breakage or split ends. In fact, whether or not hair is color-treated, you can cause the most damage by rough handling or forcing out tangles and snarls while the hair is damp.

Conditioning

To get your hair really glowing, it is very important to give your color-treated hair a conditioning or remoisturing rinse after every shampoo. I can compare this to moisturizing your skin after washing it to maintain natural oils and a healthy-looking glow.

When conditioning, it's important to remember that you don't have to condition the entire head of hair every time you shampoo. Focus in on the area of your hair that needs conditioning the most—the very ends. This is the last part of the hair shaft to get any of the natural oils from the scalp, especially if the hair is long. So, to help replenish the ends, simply work the conditioner over the surface of the hair, never throughout the hair and into the scalp area.

Color-treated (or any chemically treated) hair also needs the replenishment of a monthly conditioning treatment pack. This is left on the entire head for about twenty minutes. For an effective monthly treatment, I highly recommend La Coupe's crème régénératrice.

You don't have to spend a great deal of money on the best

Once a month, give your hair a luxurious, deep-conditioning treatment.

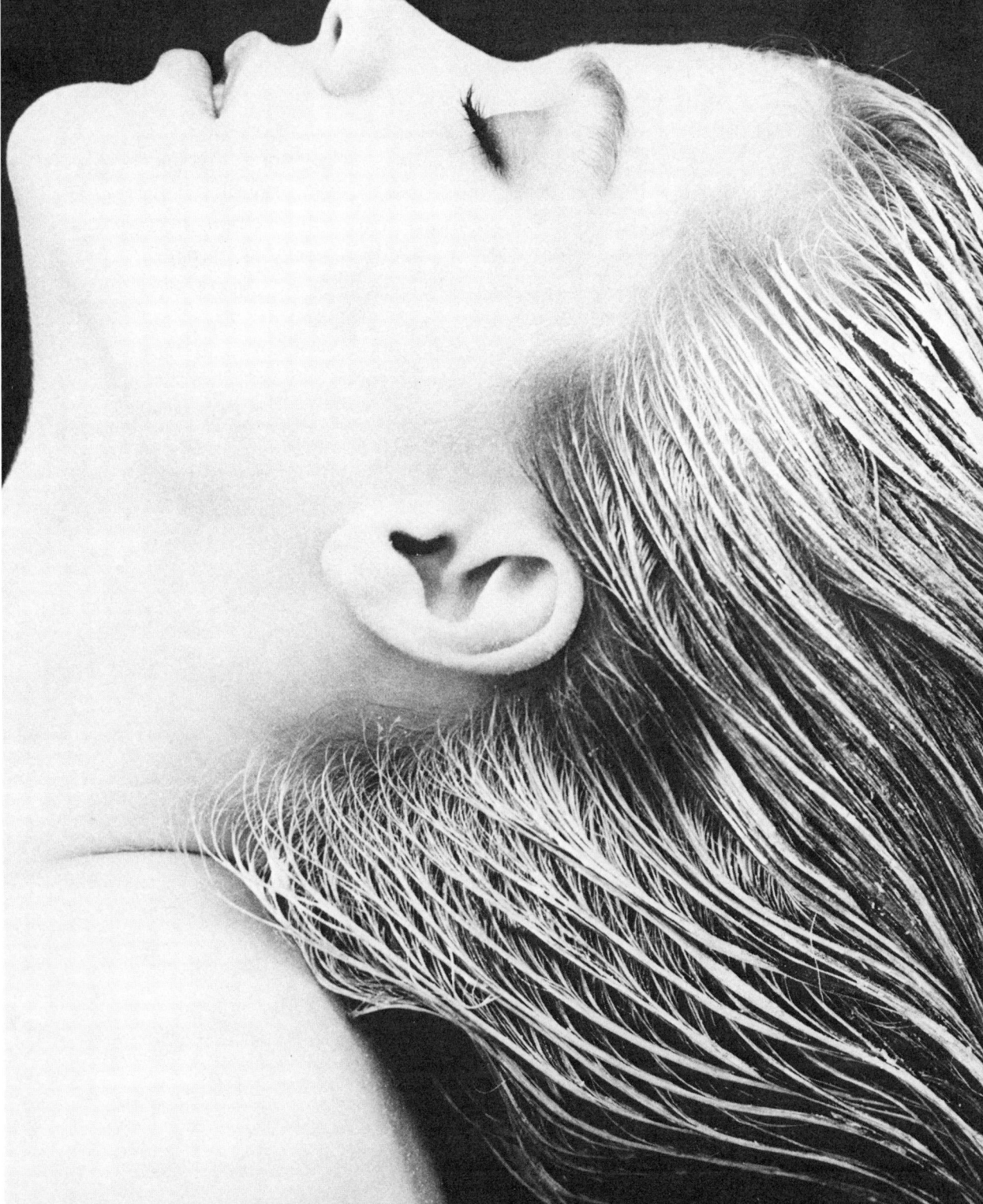

and most expensive conditioning treatments. Today, most products contain similar ingredients and therefore do the same good things for your hair. In fact, commercial conditioners are so good for your hair they almost sound good enough to eat. Your hair can enjoy the enriching benefits of everything from silk and collagen proteins to vitamins like panthenol (vitamin B) to other nurturing ingredients like wheat germ, jojoba, and even avocado oils.

Generally, I recommend a daily conditioner with a detangling quality that makes hair easier to comb. For fine hair, choose a liquid form of conditioner because it rinses out easily and leaves no film. For hair that is thick, coarse, or curly a heavy cream conditioner is your best bet; this type of hair is more porous and tends to look dry. Cream conditioners will soften and relax coarse hair to reflect maximum luster. For monthly conditioning, I recommend heat treatments in thick cream or hot oil tubes.

Regardless of the form or brand, all conditioners require a thorough rinsing. This will ensure healthy, shiny hair with no dull film remaining.

Special At-Home Recipes

To be very truthful, it's hard to beat the effectiveness of modern haircare products for keeping hair in maximum condition with minimum effort. As I have mentioned earlier, the scientists have done all the hard thinking and product testing for us—they *know* it works.

But there are times when we feel like whipping up some of our own "natural" at-home recipes to give our hair a special treatment and our senses a real treat. Like the old-fashioned vinegar or beer rinses our grandmothers used, there are many at-home blends that really do condition our hair—plus, they are just plain fun to use.

For high luster and bright highlights try my special at-home concoctions that are tried and true methods for conditioning and refreshing haircolor.

Chamomile Color Brightener Steep one-quarter cup of chamomile in a quart of boiling water. Strain off the liquid and let it cool. Use it as a final rinse after shampooing to add brightness and accentuate highlights in blond hair. *Do not rinse it off!* Leave it there to add strength to your hair. It's a great tonic for your scalp as well.

Almond Oil Rinse Almond oil makes a great conditioner for any hair. Be sparing in the amount you use (about one teaspoonful) and then shampoo well and carefully to get rid of all the excess oil. You want the look it gives your hair, not an almond film.

Apricot Wash This smells and feels as yummy as it sounds. A few drops of oil of apricot makes a fine conditioner for the hair. Use the same caution as for almond oil. Shampoo several times after rubbing the oil into your hair and scalp; it can leave a film and cause your hair to cling together.

Avocado Richness Oil of avocado adds luster and richness as part of any shampoo regimen. Don't be concerned about smelling like a salad. Just wash the hair thoroughly after each application.

Coconut Delight If you've ever used any of the suntan oils that contain coconut oil, you'll appreciate its tropical aroma. It's absolutely heaven for the nose. After applying the oil, do make sure to wash and rinse the hair thoroughly or your hair strands will cling together and look greasy. When properly applied, the results, smell, and overall feeling of this treatment make the extra trouble worthwhile.

Wheat Germ Glow Vitamin E, in large quantities, tends to make hair grow, so the story goes. Wheat germ oil, which is rich in vitamin E, makes a good conditioner, but like all the other oils it makes hair cling together and needs a good washing after each application.

Lemon Squeeze This is a refreshing rinse for blondes, both natural and lightened. It's especially helpful for the lightened blonde as lightened hair tends to be more porous and thus can cling to its neighbor. A lemon squeeze rinse not only refreshes the hair, but it also separates each strand. It's easy to make and fun to use. Squeeze three lemons, strain the seeds, and mix the juice with one pint of water. Pour it through your hair several times, then rinse. Your hair will look and feel brighter and fresher for the experience. If your hair is exceptionally oily, add one teaspoon of salt to the rinse.

Nature's Mix Try this one the next time you don't have time for a complete shampooing. Cornmeal, alone or mixed with wheat bran and orris root in equal parts, makes a great dry brush-through shampoo. Use it on a section at a time; shake a small amount of the mixture on a section of hair, brush through well, and move on to the next section. Try it . . . it really works.

Protein Whip With Eggs and Yogurt Here's one where, if you don't like the product for your hair, you can always eat it. After shampooing, use the following mixture as a conditioning treatment: one egg white, beaten well until fluffy; fold this into one-half cup of plain yogurt. Leave this mixture on your hair for 10 minutes; comb through and rinse out thoroughly. It will add fullness and luster to your hair.

Dairy Drink Here's plain yogurt again, but this time it's mixed with a bit of grated lemon rind. If your hair is short you'll only need about a teaspoon of each. Long hair may require two or three times the amount. Rub the mixture into your hair after shampooing, pulling it through all the hairs. The yogurt protein will help nourish sun-dried or chemically lightened hair. The lemon rind adds sparkle and luster.

Vinegar and Mint Tonic I know this doesn't sound as glamorous as some of the others, but, frankly, there's nothing glamorous about dandruff. An old-fashioned vinegar tonic with mint for your hair works as well today as it ever did. Add one cup of mint leaves to one cup of white vinegar and two cups of water. Boil slowly for 10 minutes. Strain the leaves and let the liquid cool on the counter. After you've shampooed, rub the tonic into your scalp. Finally, rinse well and condition.

Rosemary Rinse Rosemary will help bring out the highlights in your beautiful brunette hair. Steep one tablespoon of rosemary in one pint of boiling water. Strain the leaves and let the liquid stand until it's cool. Then use it as a final rinse after shampooing. *Don't* rinse it out afterward.

Good Ole Vinegar Rinse Two tablespoons of white vinegar in a quart of warm water will add shine, luster and softness to your freshly washed hair. It's simple, quick, and extremely inexpensive.

The New Freedom of Modern Haircolor

It's really important to realize that coloring your hair doesn't mean you must "baby" it as women did years ago. Modern

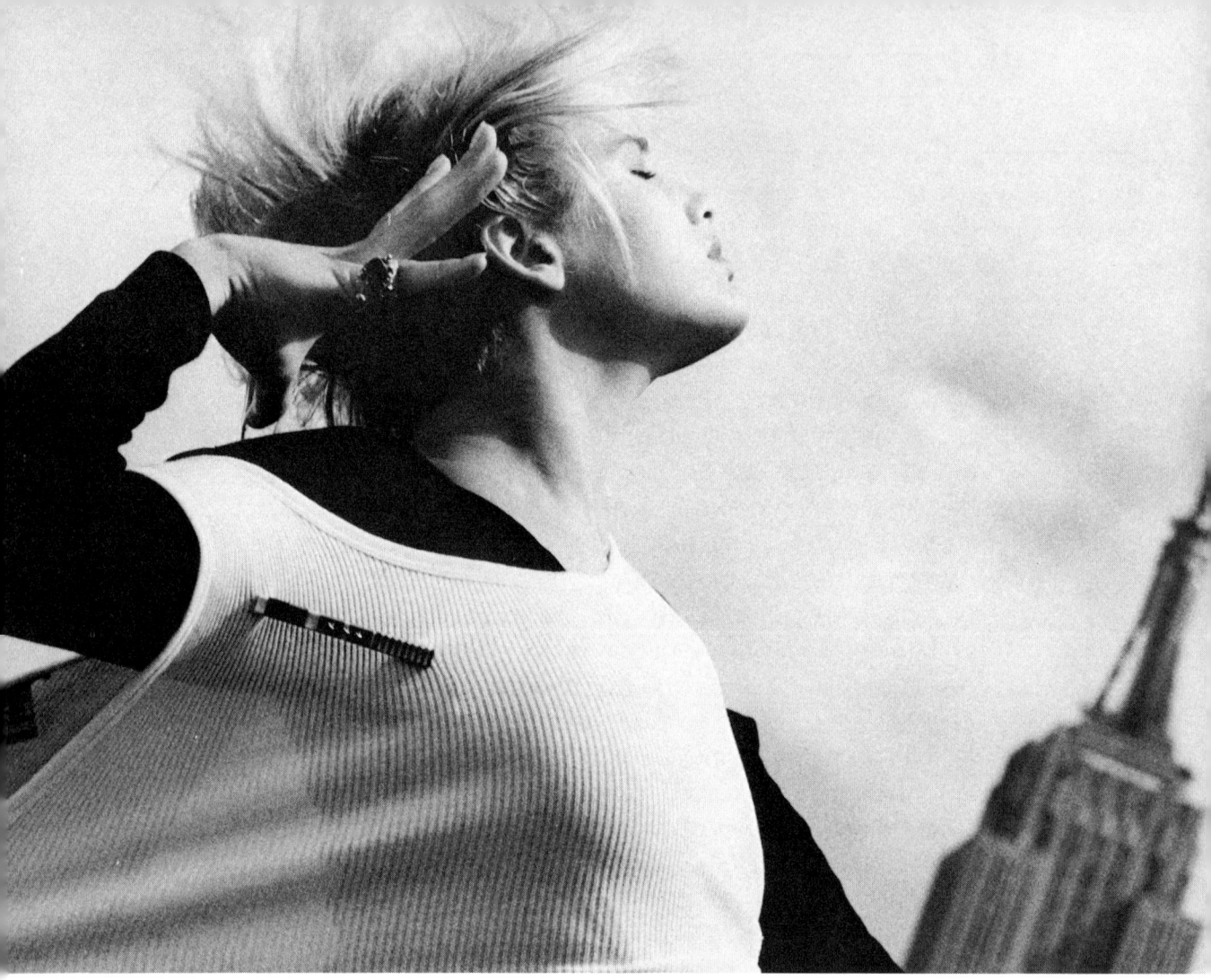

haircolor is not only easy now to do but it's even easier to maintain. You can forget about your hair; just enjoy it.

No doubt you still have some questions about how your hair or haircolor may be affected under certain conditions and it's important for you to have those answers.

First of all, you don't have to go around wearing a hat in the sun for the rest of your life. That was *yesterday's* haircoloring need. If you didn't wear a cover of some sort, your haircolor would fade. Today, we have learned that the sun actually can improve upon our haircoloring. It adds a bit of brightness and

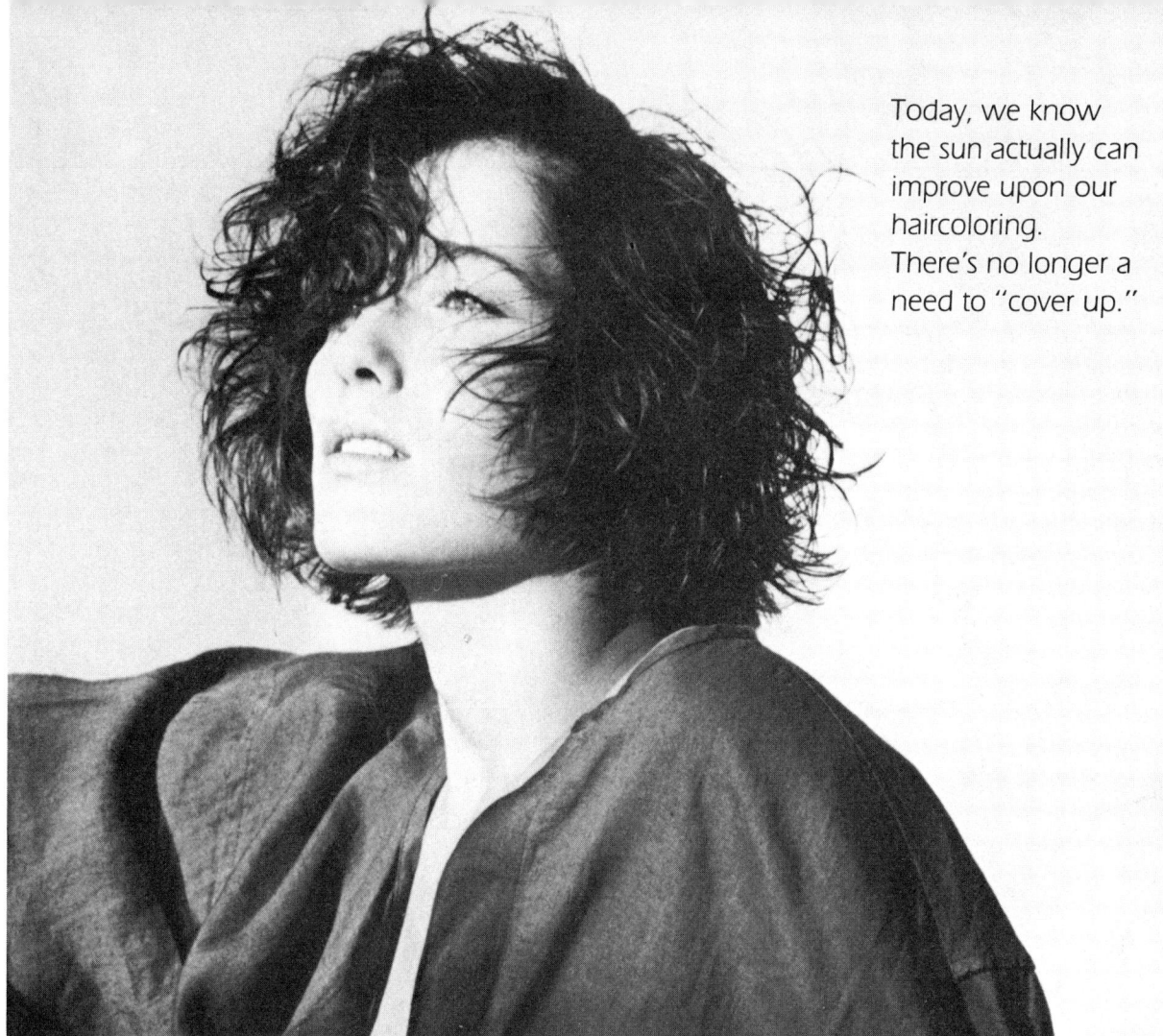

Today, we know the sun actually can improve upon our haircoloring. There's no longer a need to "cover up."

additional highlights that accent great color. So, if you color your hair, go out in the sun and enjoy it; there's no need to hide. Think of the sun as a wonderful suntan for your hair as well as for your skin.

Chlorine and salt water raised havoc with yesterday's haircolor, especially with redheads and blondes. But, today, redheads and blondes can be assured of rich, vibrant color with reasonable use of a chlorinated pool or salt water. I say *reasonable,* because too much of either or both will alter haircolor faster than you may wish.

To delay this from happening, I suggest smoothing conditioner on your hair (especially the ends) before jumping into the pool or the ocean. This will really protect the hair and keep anything harsh from penetrating the hair shaft.

In fact, wearing conditioner on your hair poolside or on the beach has become quite fashionable. After applying conditioner, just mold your hair into a sleek shape. You'll be wearing the "wet look" and be very chic in the process of protecting your hair.

Many clients ask me if they can perm their hair if they color it. Yes—again due to modern product technology.

I always recommend doing your *perm first, and your color one week later.* This allows your permanent to "take" and neutralize over several days, and then receive color evenly, one week later. Perm and color can coexist beautifully on one head of hair thanks to modern products that condition while they perform their specific magic.

Another frequent question has to do with thermal or heat-producing styling appliances like blow-dryers, electric rollers, and curling irons. Will these affect haircolor?

It's not the haircolor alone that will be affected by these types of appliances; the general condition of the hair must be monitored. Recall that I stressed the importance of handling color-treated hair gently—no tugging, pulling, and yanking, especially when wet. Be careful how you handle your hair while you're styling with thermal appliances. Too much heat, *too close* to the hair (while blow-drying) is not good for any type of hair. It will dry the hair and encourage the ends to split or create dry areas that you don't want.

Be reasonable with your hair when using a heat-producing source. Too much of anything will have some negative effect.

Chapter 7

"Dull-to-Dazzling" Haircolor Makeovers

Every woman has a natural beauty all her own. But there are times when an objective, interested observer (like a professional) can take one look at a woman and know there's *a lot* more to her than meets the eye.

I think every woman's looks should reflect her true personality. And haircolor is the most effective vehicle to make this happen—more so than new makeup, new clothes, and losing ten pounds. The right haircolor will wake up everything about you—think about what may be hiding behind your dull hair and pale complexion.

So, do you want to look okay or fabulous? Here are some "dull to dazzling" makeovers that will illustrate just what haircolor can do for you.

Gabrielle

 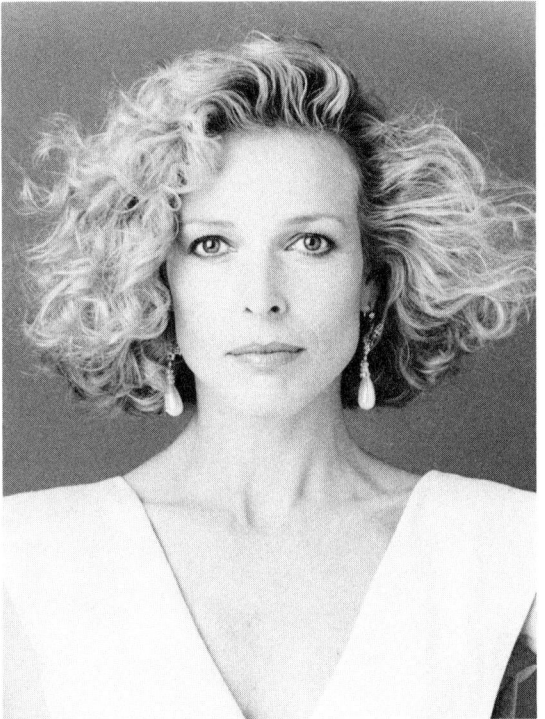

A professional model with Ford, Gabrielle is considered the classic beauty—high cheekbones, beautiful pale skin, and golden blond hair. To maintain her sunny-looking haircolor, I added allover fine highlighting that makes her sparkle in both her professional and personal life.

LOUIS' PERSONAL FORMULA

Before:
Dull blond.

Formula:
Allover fine highlighting for the brightest blond look; Clairol's Light Effects for Blondes.

After:
Beautiful shining blond hair.

Toni

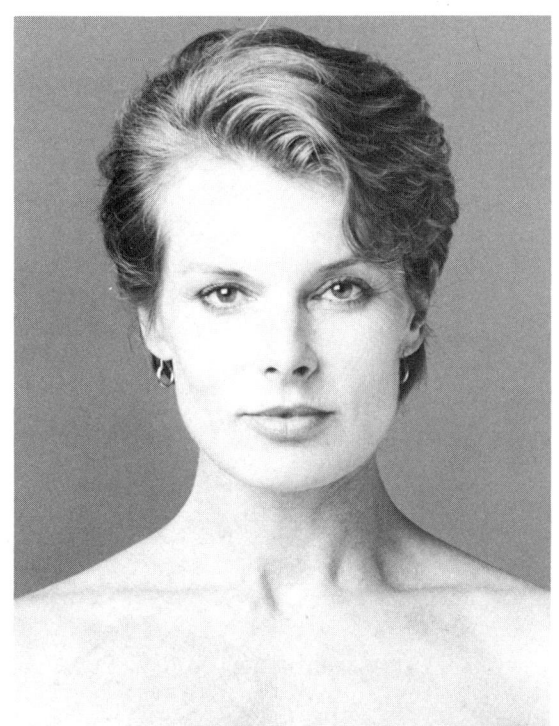 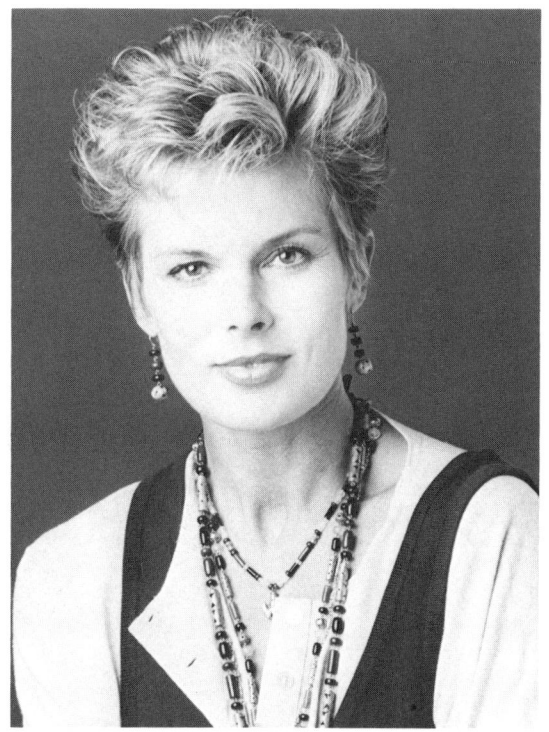

I think Toni gives her fullest to everything she does. She works hard, plays hard, and succeeds at just about everything she attempts. I call her a total pro. A professional model and author, Toni comes from a whole family of beauties. She needed an accent of color to carry through her natural chic from head to toe.

LOUIS' PERSONAL FORMULA

Before:

Light brown short hair that needed some accent and softness.

Formula:

The pretty "up cut" was accented with warm golden highlights, especially within the top section where hair was longer; Clairol's Special Effects for Brown.

Result:

Lighter tones throughout hair—an excellent example of how cut and color can work together.

Lynn

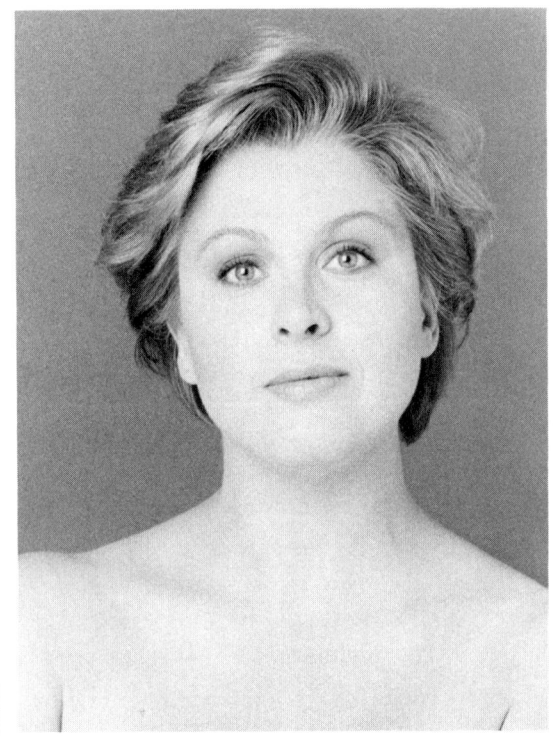 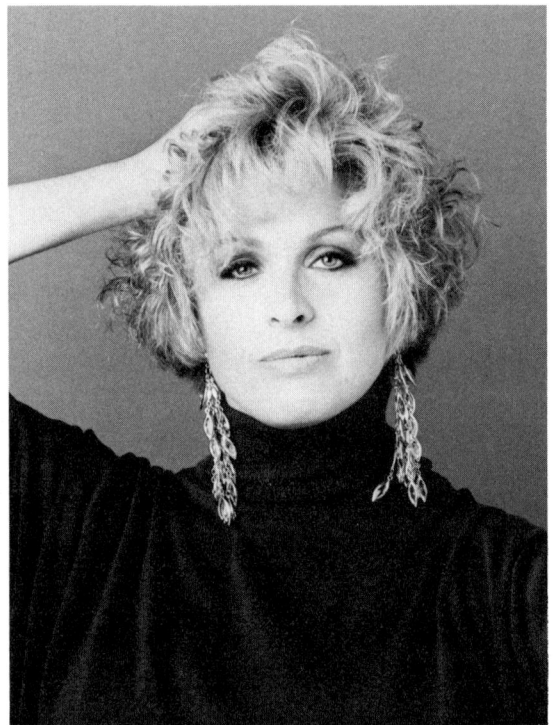

Lynn is definitely a bold, single Manhattan woman. Although she is not a shy person, her appearance projected a rather quiet and reserved demeanor. Lynn needed a brighter haircolor that conveyed her bright, aggressive personality.

LOUIS' PERSONAL FORMULA

Before:
Mousy light brown hair.

Formula:
Flaxen blond permanent color, plus highlights to frame the face and accent the cut; Clairol's Frost 'n Tip.

After:
Pretty warm blond with highlights.

Heidi

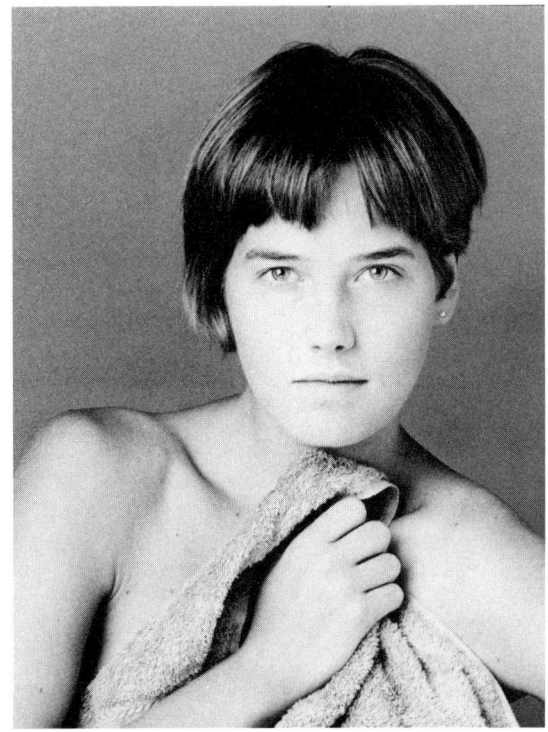 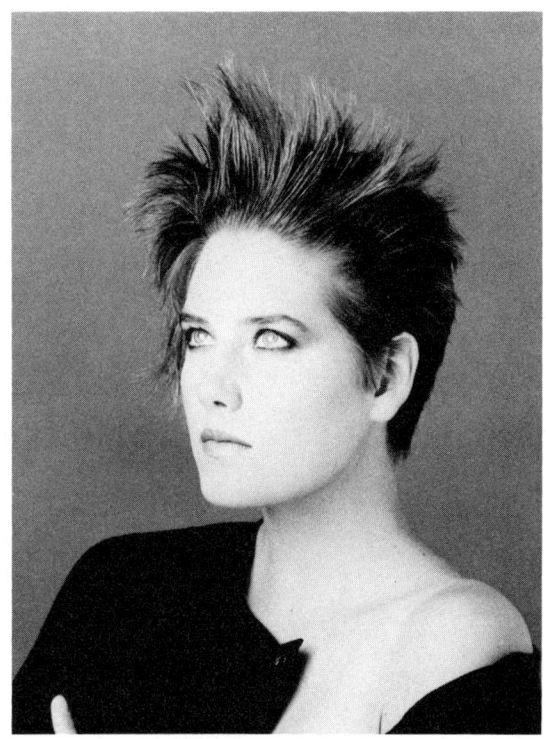

Heidi can be described as a wonderful contradiction of personalities—simple and sweet by day, electric and tempestuous at night. She has a fabulous cut that is as contemporary and creative as she is. Heidi needed color to accent her cut and to play up her wonderful mix of personal qualities.

LOUIS' PERSONAL FORMULA

Before:

Rather ordinary light brown hair.

Formula:

The tipping technique was used to outline or silhouette the style and add some color interest and accent.

Result:

Brown hair came alive with beautiful golden lights.

Alisha

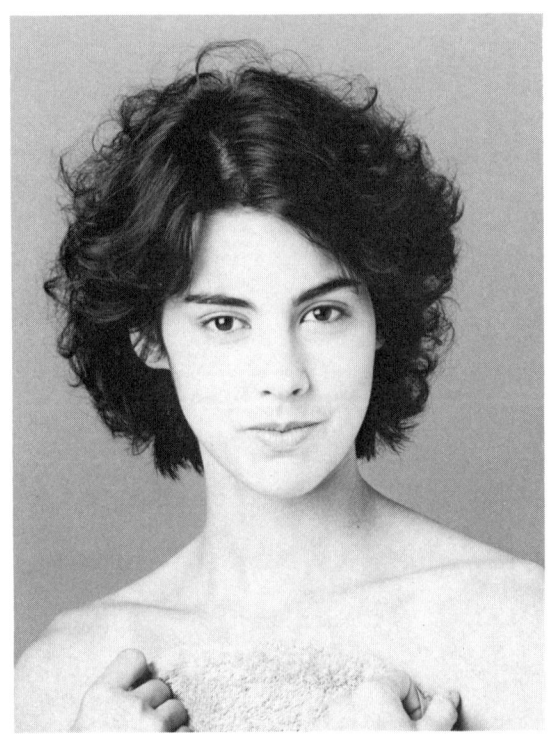 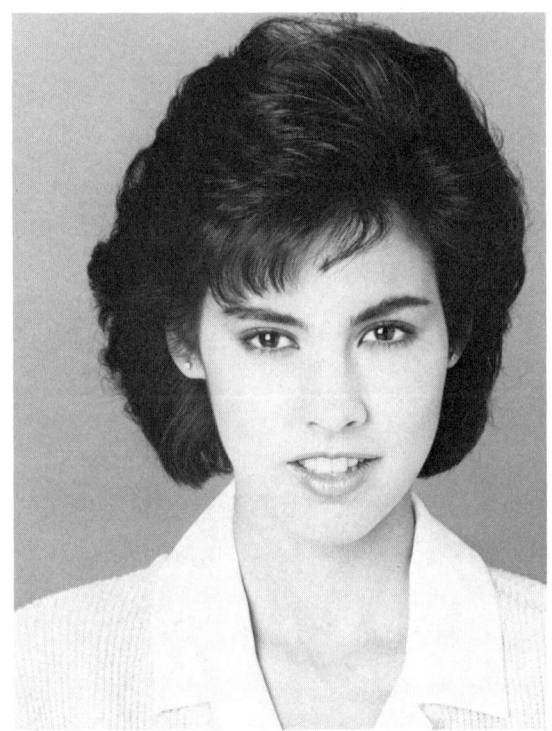

Alisha has an exotic, striking appearance that she inherited from her Indian father and beautiful mother, of course. She is also a successful young actress who must look fabulous for auditions. Her haircolor failed to portray her best image—it looked dry, dull, and very uninspiring for such an inspired young woman.

LOUIS' PERSONAL FORMULA

Before:

Blah brown hair that looked dry and limp.

Formula:

Medium warm brown semipermanent color slightly lighter than natural color; Clairol's Loving Care.

Results:

Rich, burnished brunette color plus shine, fullness, and better texture.

Kathy

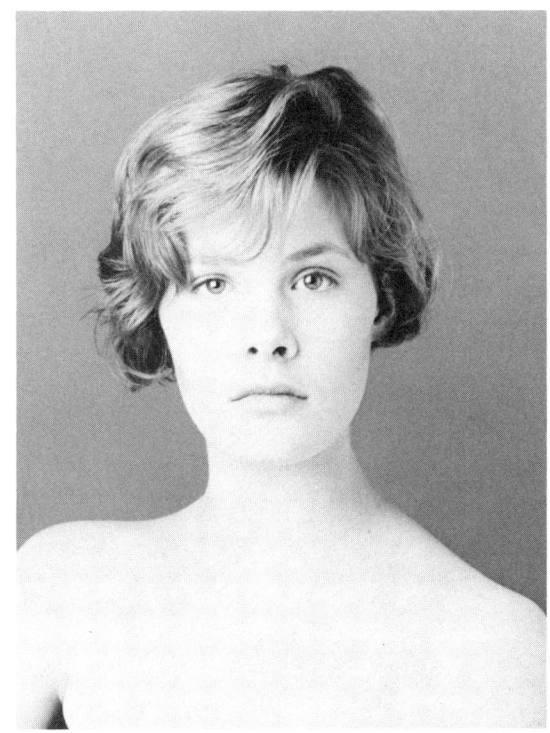 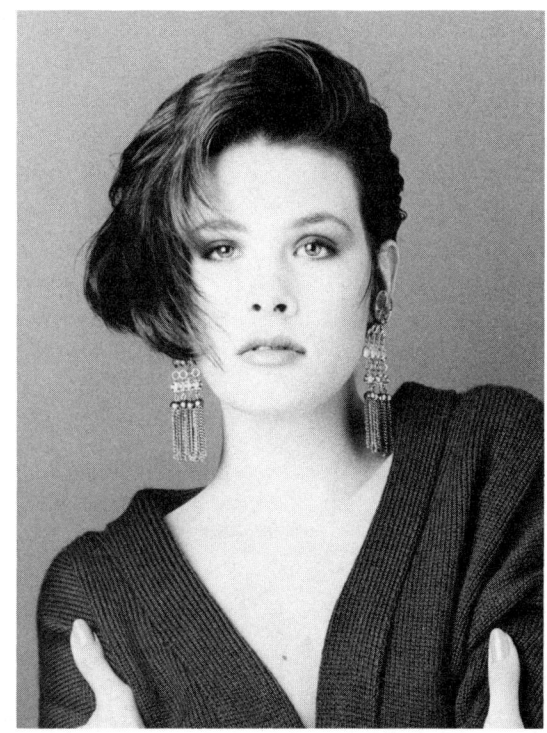

Kathy is a young, outdoorsy woman from Colorado. When she moved to New York, she wanted to citify her fashion image. She wanted to look more sophisticated and was very enthusiastic about getting her image updated.

LOUIS' PERSONAL FORMULA

Before:
"No-color" hair.

Formula:
One-step (no-peroxide) permanent color in a rich copper shade to add warmth and vibrance.

Result:
Rich coppery auburn hair.

Suzanne

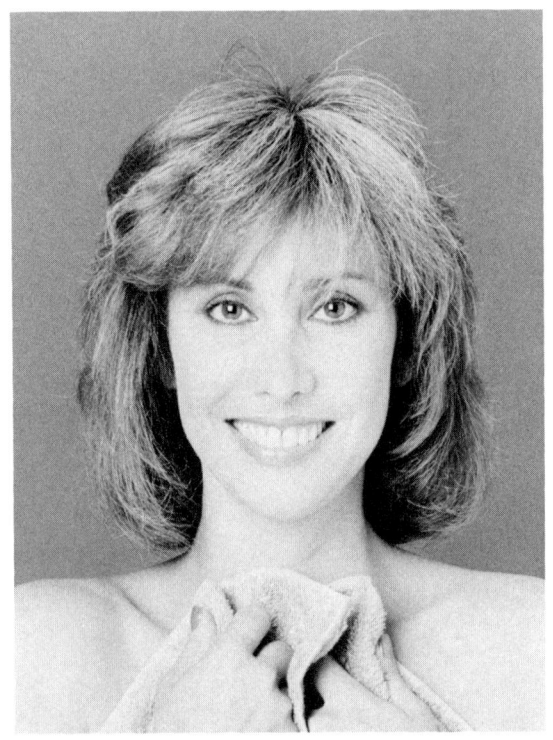 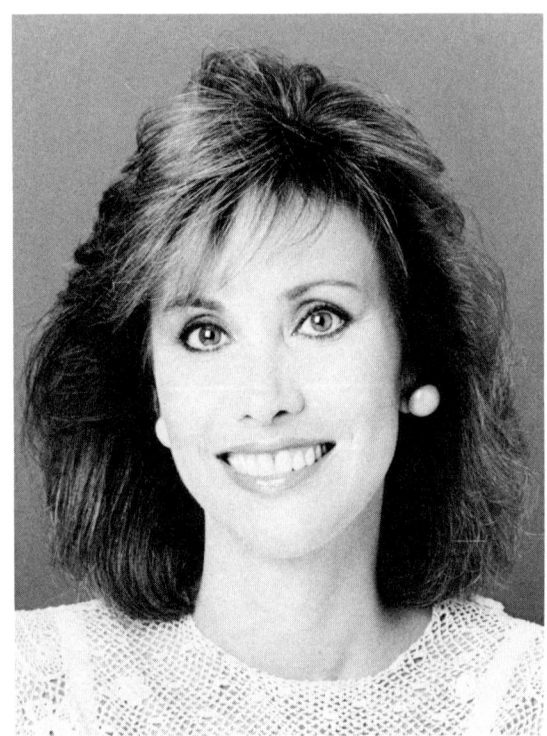

Suzanne is one of my favorite clients. She needed a dynamic color change to match her dynamic personality. The young wife of an executive, a new mother with a keen interest in the communications field, Suzanne was not ready to accept that dulling, graying hair she began to notice.

LOUIS' PERSONAL FORMULA

Before:

Light brown hair starting to gray (about 30 percent). Hair looked dull and so did skin tones and eye color.

Formula:

A light golden brown semipermanent color.

Result:

Gray hairs turned into natural-looking highlights. Allover base color became warmer and brighter.

Janelle

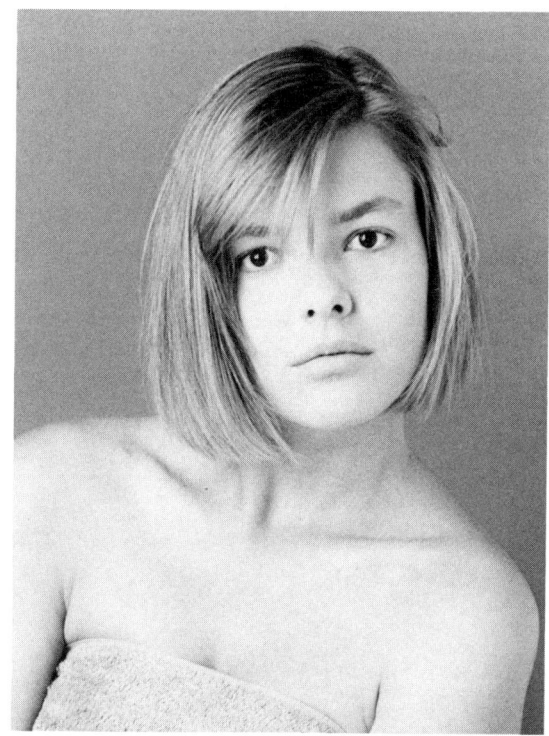 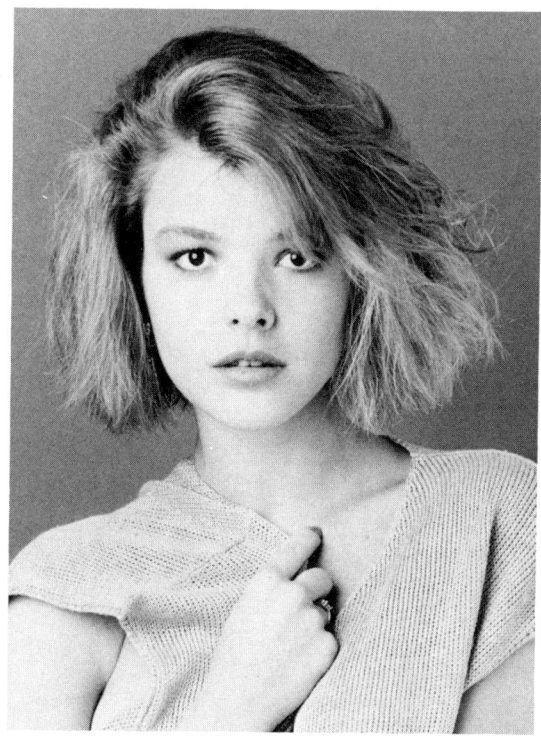

Janelle is an aspiring young actress from the Midwest. She has a natural beauty that only needed a pinch of color to accent her skin tones and eye color. It was just the right touch to put Manhattan sparkle into her Midwestern blond hair.

LOUIS' PERSONAL FORMULA

Before:
Dull blond.

Formula:
Hair painting done over surface of hair just as the sun would lighten it.

Result:
The look of a summer of sun in the middle of winter.

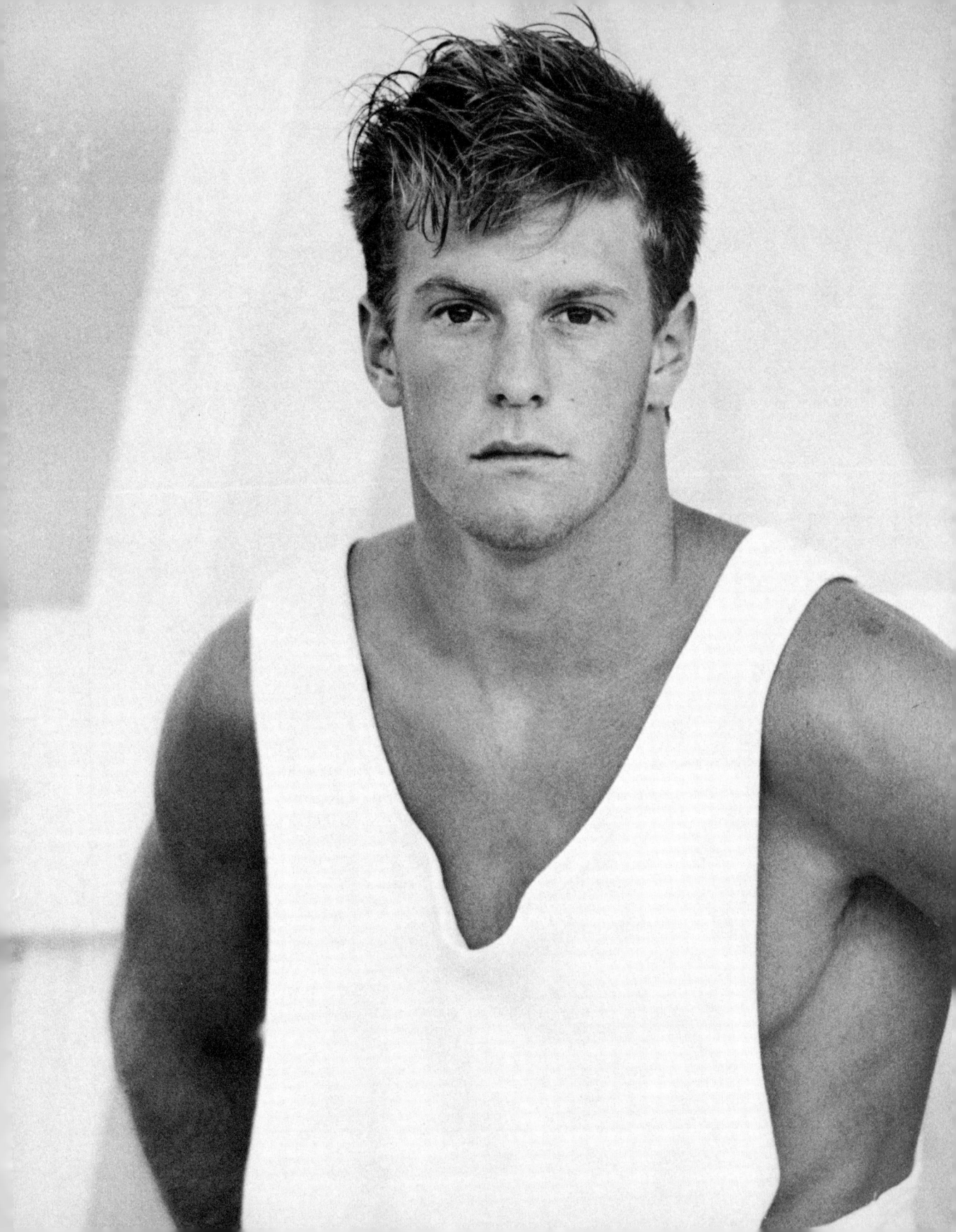

Chapter 8

Haircolor for Men

The Modern Haircolor Revolution

Executives, college students, professional athletes, and even construction workers—everyone is coloring their hair these days.

Haircoloring is no longer something for men to think about in the future. It's here and it's now! Men already are coloring their hair in droves because it's fun, easy, and it makes them look terrific.

Women are an important part of the men's haircolor revolution. Because they already know the benefits of modern haircolor, women are encouraging their husbands and boyfriends to try the latest products and shades. In fact, in many cases, they are doing the man's color at home!

One part of the revolution that has not yet hit the eighties is a good selection of haircolor products especially for men. Not only are few items manufactured, but those that are available possess many faults. Some of the most harmless-looking coloring products—like those clear liquids that "gradually" deepen and darken hair—can actually leave a greenish cast after several applications. This is because they contain metallic salts which can cause hair to go "ashy" or green. For this reason, I always recommend women's products for men. Not only is there a vast selection, but you'll find even some "token" men appearing on the boxes. So, don't feel totally ignored.

When to Think About Coloring Your Hair

Most men, like women, begin to think about changing their haircolor when they start to gray. First the gray strands creep in around the hairline and men always try to pull them out or hope they won't be noticed; but when those grays grow in faster than we wish, it's time for haircolor!

As hair starts to gray, our appearance can take on a dull look. One glance in the mirror may show faded skin tones, dulling eyes, and the lack of that certain sparkle we had a few years ago. Haircolor can bring back our youthful image and turn that dull gray into a natural-looking blend of lights and tones.

Interestingly enough, the younger generation is using color, too. Guys in their teens and their twenties are flocking to the haircolor shelves to buy spray-in lighteners that create highlights in and out of the sun. One of the most popular brands for younger guys who love what I call the beach-bum look is

Clairol's A Little Sun or A Lot of Sun, actually aimed at teenage girls.

One of the traditional times men rethink their total fashion image and, therefore, their haircolor is when a major job promotion is due. This occurs to men usually in their thirties. Suddenly they realize they have dressed the same way for about ten years and have probably worn the same haircut since high school. This is definitely the time to enhance blah brown or mousy blond hair, or to add some highlights at the sideburns or at the top of the head for an uplifting effect. Let's face it—when you look your best, you feel your best, and those are the guys that get the promotions.

Popular Haircolor Options

One of the easiest ways for men to create subtle highlights exactly where they want them is hair painting. All you do is use a fine brush to apply a creamy lightening mixture along the natural waves or other areas of the cut that need accenting. It all comes in an easy-to-use complete at-home hair painting kit.

Here's a helpful guide for placing your highlights: Just think of where you get natural highlights in the summer. Try to duplicate these areas, using your brush to do the sun's handiwork.

Semipermanent colors are a great way of turning your grays into highlights that blend into a natural background. You can also use the semipermanents to enhance your own color while adding body and shine to hair.

Younger men are using color gels to add shine and shape to their cuts, plus an interesting "reflective" color quality that looks great under party lights. This is haircolor with which men can have fun at night; just wash it out the next morning.

I usually create a "surfer lights" look on the younger men at my salon. I lighten or darken selected strands at the temples and on top for either a highlighted look or a tone-on-tone effect (light brown strands against dark brown). It's kind of fun to look like you live in Malibu even though you reside in New York, Chicago, or St. Louis.

Finally, I think the special shampoos and temporary rinses designed to enhance gray are wonderful. Some of them reduce the yellow tone that gray hair often develops; others simply make gray hair brighter, more shiny and very pearlescent.

Haircolor Q & A

For the millions of men who have never before colored their hair or never even thought about it until now, here are some helpful answers to questions I most often receive from male clients.

Q. *I wouldn't know where or how to begin coloring my hair; I would be "all thumbs." But I do like the thought of having my hair look like I just spent a summer in the sun. What should I do?*

A. If you feel totally insecure about your own coloring ability, I definitely recommend going to a styling salon and asking the colorist to explain the technique of highlighting. Perhaps you have a lady in your life who is quite adept at coloring her own hair—she would probably love to color yours! The whole experience is sure to be lots of fun and you'll love the results—highlights you never dreamed of having in the middle of winter!

Q. *My hair never looked better. I think it's because my stylist permed a couple of problem areas that always went flat or fell in my face. Now I've got the body I want in my hair but the color looks flat. Can I have both perm and color in my hair?*

A. Yes, you can have *both* without that dry look you may be associating with chemically treated hair. I would recommend a professional haircolorist for you. He or she will work carefully with your hair texture and probably also recommend a conditioning routine to keep your hair looking shiny. *Note:* A good rule to follow is to have your perm done first, and then the color *one week later or longer.*

Q. *Will I have roots if I color my hair all over?*

A. Not if you choose a shade very close to or slightly lighter than your natural color. I recommend semipermanent color which will last four to six shampoos and then fade away if you decide not to continue your color applications.

Q. *What's the best product for coloring gray? I am now about 80 percent gray.*

A. Permanent color will give you the most effective, longest-lasting coverage of gray hair. I hate to say it, but the best haircolor choices for you are in the women's section of color products—like Miss Clairol or Nice 'n Easy.

I do recommend strongly, however, that you begin covering your gray with a semipermanent color like Loving Care. This will give you a feeling for what haircolor can offer, yet offer you the option of not continuing or trying something else if you're not pleased with the results.

Perhaps a female friend should join you in the women's haircolor section to make you feel more comfortable in your choice of haircolor.

Q. *If I color my hair, do I neeed to use any special conditioners?*

A. You don't need to use "special" conditioners; they're all pretty much alike. What's important is *how often* you condition your hair. I recommend a light instant "moisturizer" once a month after shampooing for an added healthy glow to hair.

How-to Haircolor Techniques

SURFER LIGHTS

This technique is the easiest, most popular way to add natural-looking highlights exactly where you want them. You can do it yourself effortlessly using Clairol's Hair Painting kit (it includes the brush). Just remember to begin with dry hair.

1   Part your hair in the desired style.

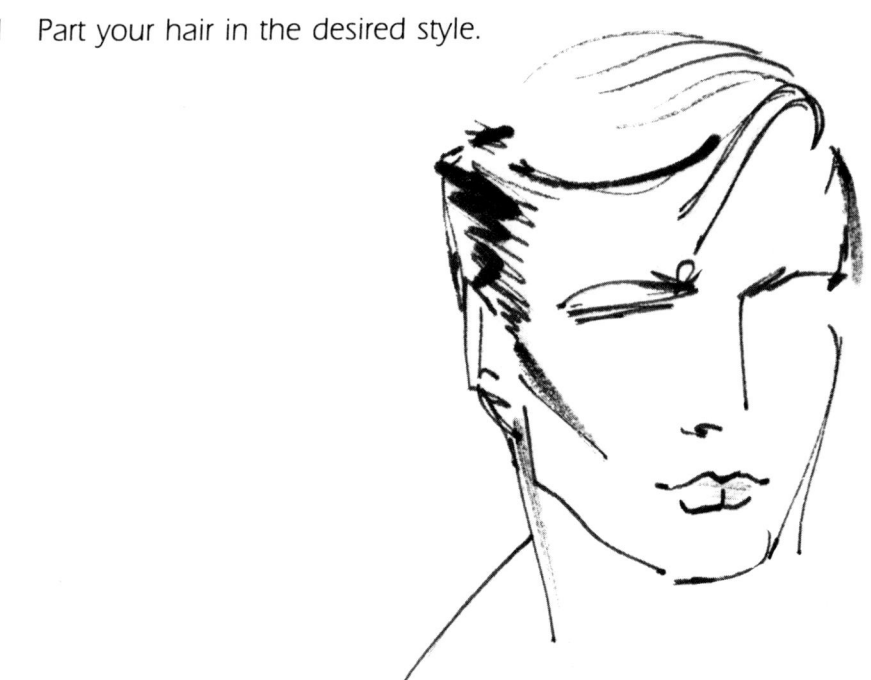

2   Put on plastic gloves.

3   Mix developer and special lightening powder in the plastic bowl enclosed.

4   Dip brush in creme mixture and apply to fine strands on the surface of the hair (where the sun lightens). Create highlights in any section you want, but be sure to take your cut into consideration—there may be areas that can be accented nicely with some highlights.

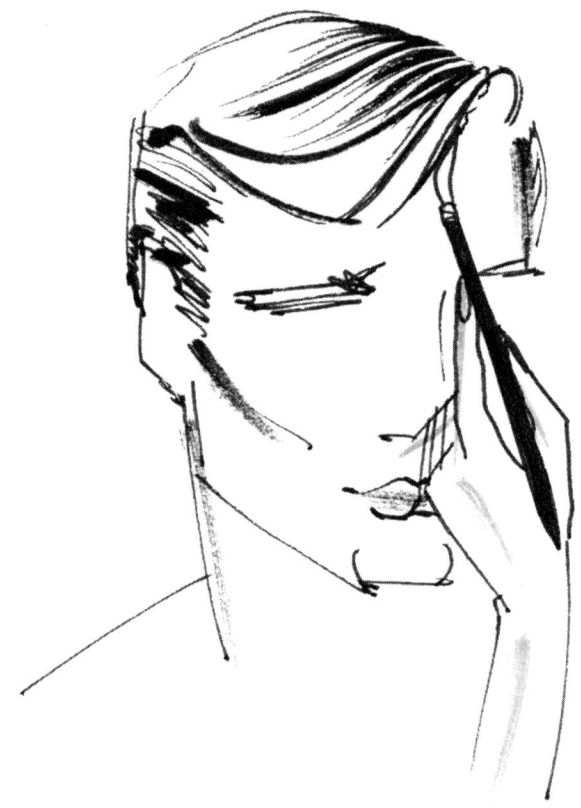

5   Leave the mixture on for the amount of time recommended in the instructions of the hair painting kit. Don't forget to *set your timer.*

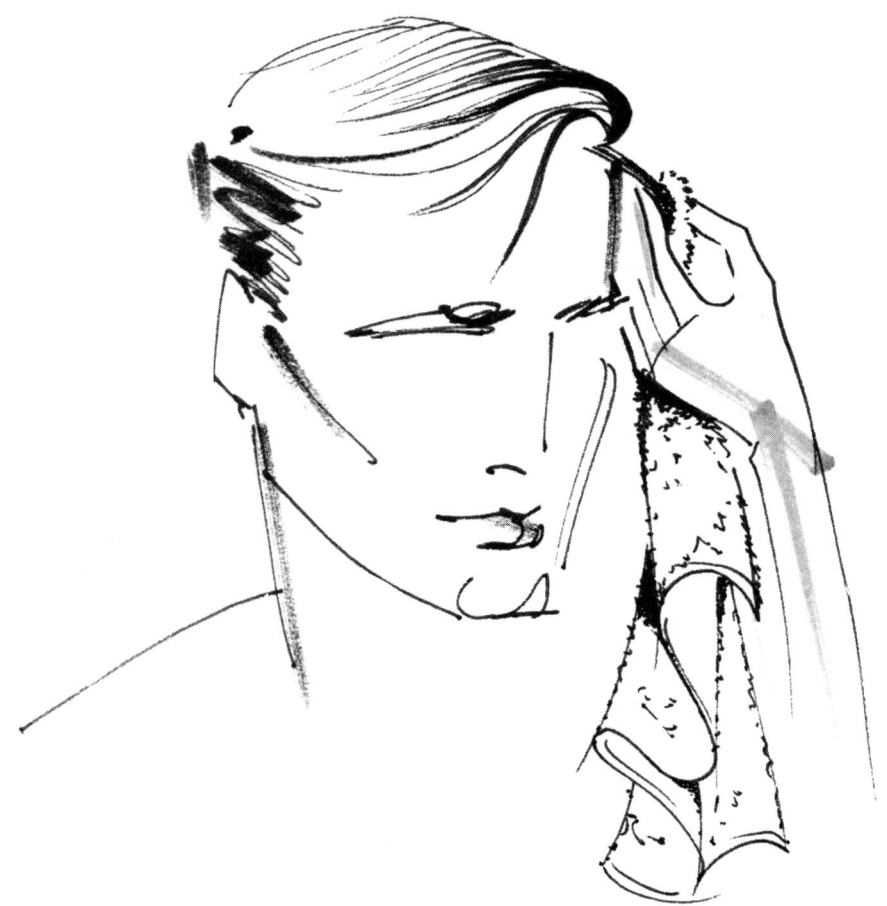

6   After five minutes, you may wish to preview the degree of color by toweling off some of the mixture on a few strands.

7   When developing time is up, and you're pleased with the degree of lightness, shampoo out mixture with the special packet of conditioning shampoo enclosed in the kit. You can use your regular shampoo, but be sure to condition your hair as well and style as usual.

BLENDING

Blending is a process that camouflages the gray in dull salt-and-pepper hair, using a semipermanent color. I recommend Clairol's Loving Care in a shade slightly lighter than your own. It actually will turn your gray strands into healthy-looking highlights. This technique requires no special sectioning of hair. Finally, the hair should be dry.

1 Put on gloves.

2 Apply cream all around the hairline to prevent color from staining skin. Adhere cotton to the cream.

3 Mix the haircolor formula in the plastic bottle following directions.

4 Squeeze small amounts of formula from bottle into the palm of your hand and lather throughout the hair.

5 Let the color develop for the length of time specified in instructions. *Set your timer.*

6 When the time is up, shampoo out; condition and style as usual.

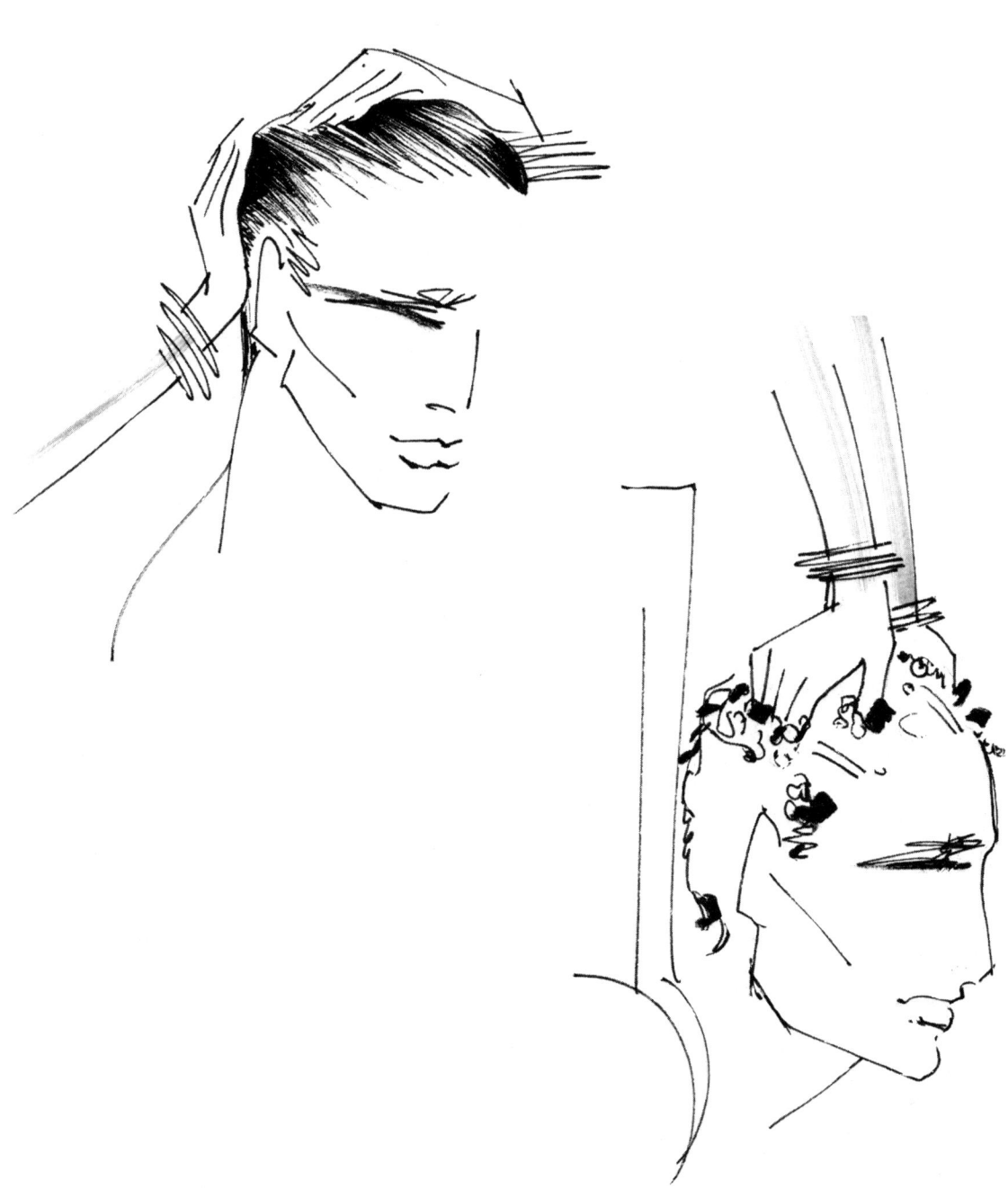

Beards, Mustaches, and Sideburns

Haircolor can be your best friend when it comes to touching up those tricky little areas where hair doesn't quite match your basic haircolor—namely, your beard, mustache, or sideburns.

What you should do is subtly blend these areas with a shade close to your own color for a cleaner, more contemporary image. Men can often look kind of "scraggly" if they have a reddish beard with brown hair, or a whitish beard with red hair, or perhaps a gray mustache and blond sideburns.

Pull it all together with haircolor for "total color blending." To begin, I suggest trying a semipermanent color that closely matches your own. Because the facial area is washed often, the semipermanent color will fade rather quickly—about two weeks after the first application. If it disappears too soon for your taste, it's time to graduate to a permanent color for longer-lasting depth of color and coverage of gray.

For touch-ups requiring accuracy in placement, I suggest using a Q-Tip or a fine brush to apply the color.

FACIAL HAIR TOUCH-UP

1. Put on gloves.

2. Mix color according to directions.

3. Apply color to the desired area with either a Q-Tip or a fine brush.

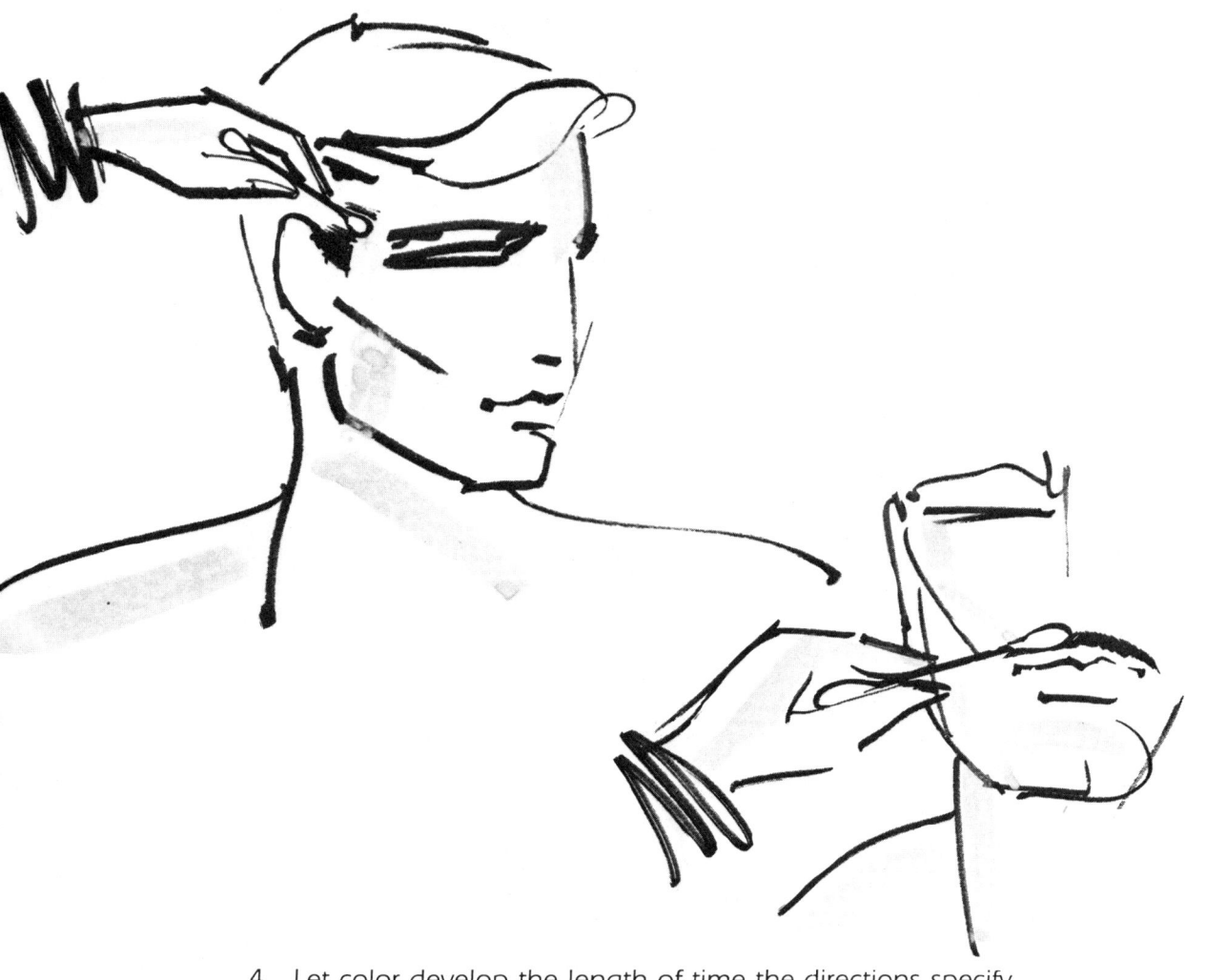

4   Let color develop the length of time the directions specify. *Set timer.* After five minutes, you may wish to preview the degree of color by toweling off some of the mixture from a few strands of hair.

5   Shampoo out color mixture and let dry as usual.

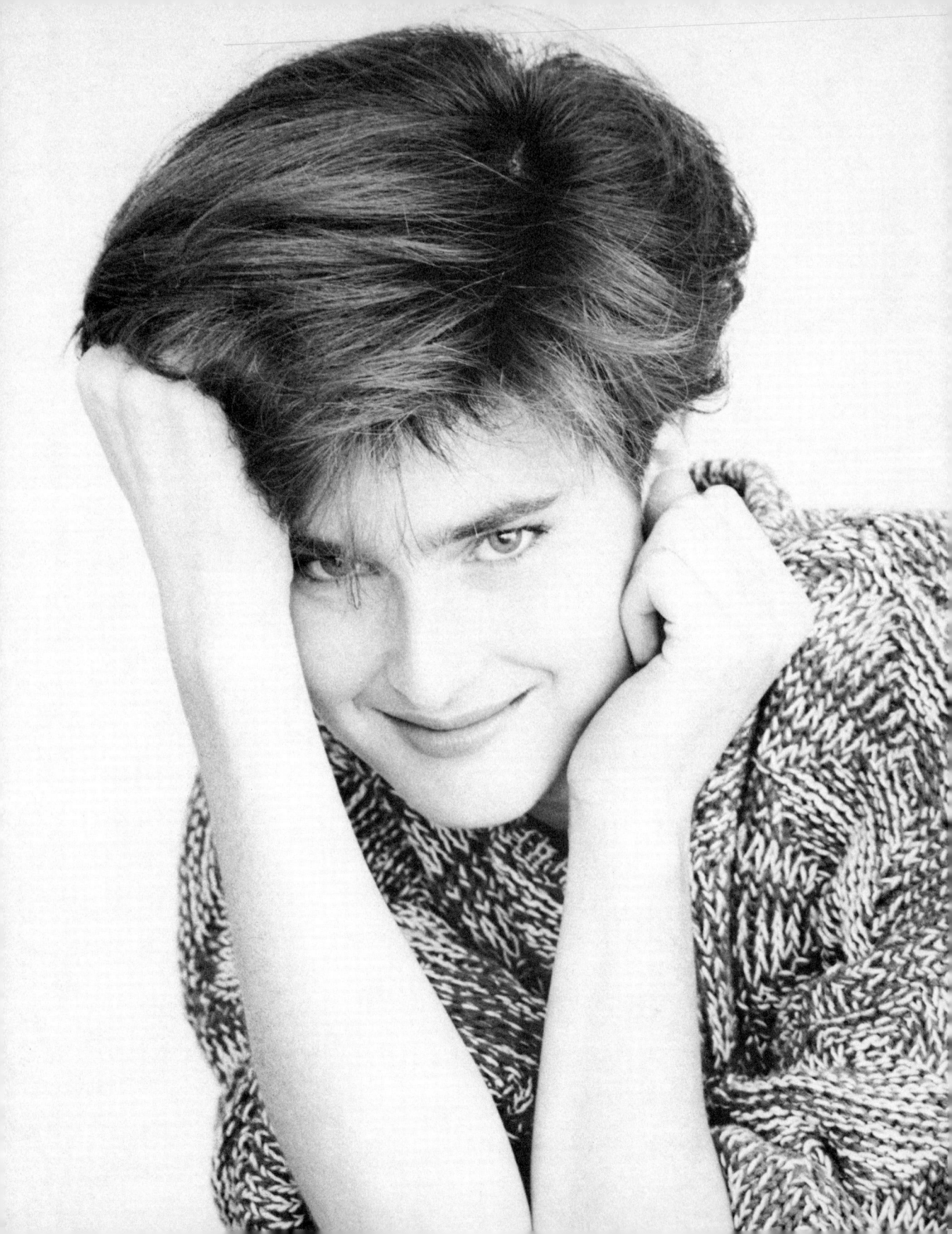

Be the Best You Can Be . . . With Haircolor

Today is the day to color your hair. Modern haircolor is something you *want* to do, no longer something you *must* do. When your color is right, your face will radiate a healthy glow. Your looks come alive, and you somehow feel *so much* better about yourself.

Once you color your hair, it's a perfect time to rethink the colors of your clothes and makeup. It may be time to introduce some interesting new shades that complement your haircolor, but rest assured that you don't have to redo your whole closet or replace all your cosmetics.

Remember that your new shade of haircolor should not be *that* different from your natural color, so you won't have to make any drastic adjustments in other areas of your life.

If you have chosen to play up the red in your hair, for example, add some copper or teal or plum tones to your wardrobe. If

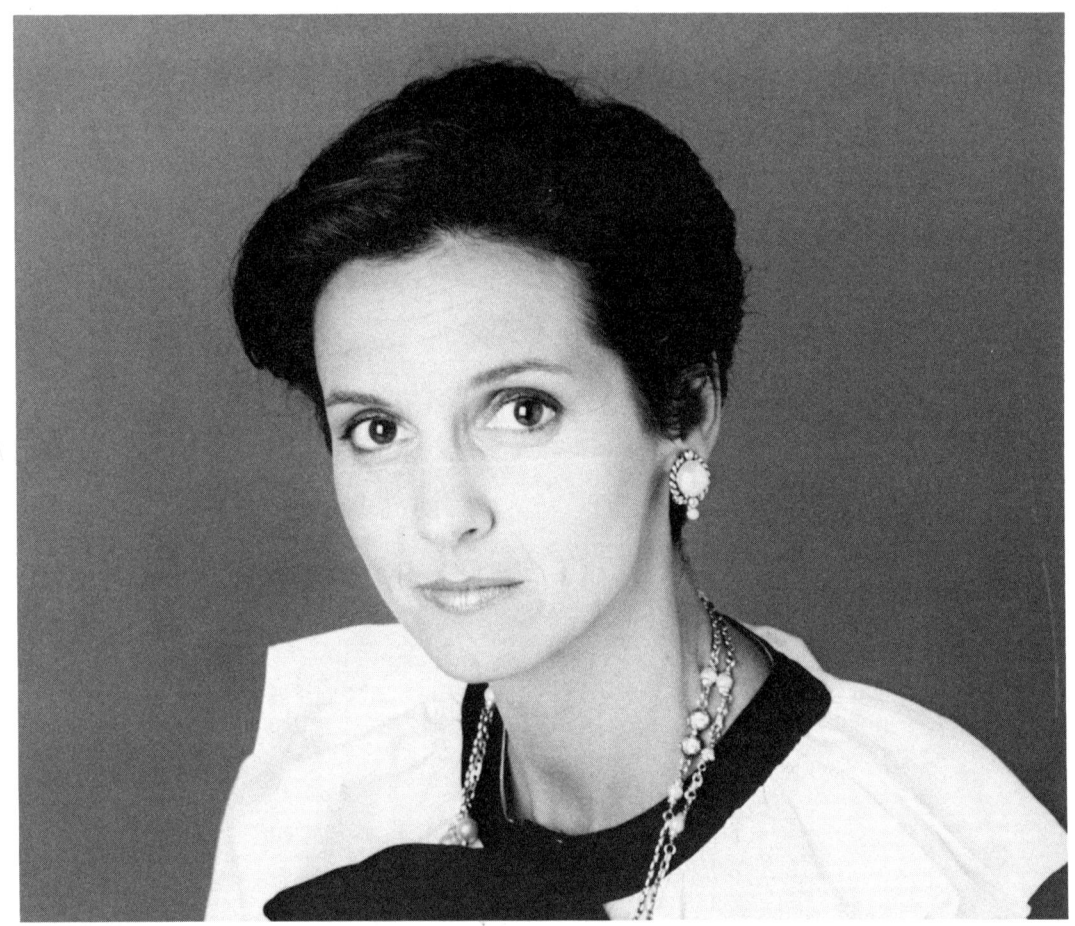

According to Harper's Bazaar *Beauty Editor Carlotta Karlson Jacobson, haircolor is a person's most important fashion accessory. It also works hand in hand with your total look.*

"Once a woman does try haircolor," says Carlotta, "she realizes how important it is to her total color balance—with her makeup, clothes, natural skin tones, etc. We really can't have one without the other."

Carlotta, a striking brunette, prefers the more temporary forms of haircolor, like the semipermanents, to enhance her rich brown hair. She believes that the woman who is thinking about coloring her hair can easily "try on" a new shade because of these great, new, more temporary products.

you have brought your brunette hair from dull to dazzling, I suggest adding some brighter colors to your closet like true reds, lemon yellows, and royal blues. Blondes who have gone more golden or more wheat-toned should add more neutrals to their wardrobe like off-whites, creams, eggshell, beiges, and grays; I call these "blonde colors" because they *always* look stunning against beautiful blond hair.

I use the same color principles when it comes to makeup. Select some new tones in your lipsticks, blushers, and eye shadows; it makes sense to get some expert opinions on the best cosmetic choices for your haircolor from the consultants at the cosmetic counter or even from a makeup artist at your salon.

To me, this feels like the end of a fabulous color consultation with a client. This is the point where I always know that my client's life is about to change and become a wonderful new experience. And it's all because she has made one simple but important decision—to color her hair and color her life.

If you're this person, I congratulate you and personally welcome you to the world of modern haircolor.